GASTRIC COOKBOOK
FOR ALL STAGES

*Quick and Easy Mouthwatering Recipes to Avoid
Weight Gain at all Stages After Bariatric Surgery*

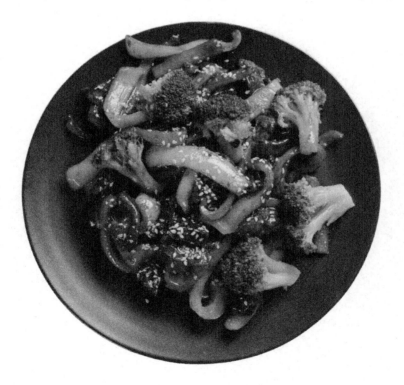

DR. SANDRA T. CADWELL

GASTRIC BYPASS COOKBOOK FOR ALL STAGES

Copyright © 2024 Dr. Sandra T. Cadwell
All rights reserved.

No part of this publication may be reproduced, distributed, or transmitted in any form or by any means, including photocopying, recording, or other electronic or mechanical methods, without the prior written permission of the publisher, except in the case of brief quotations embodied in critical reviews and certain other noncommercial uses permitted by copyright law.

This cookbook is a work of non-fiction. The recipes, tips, and advice provided are based on the author's experiences and research.

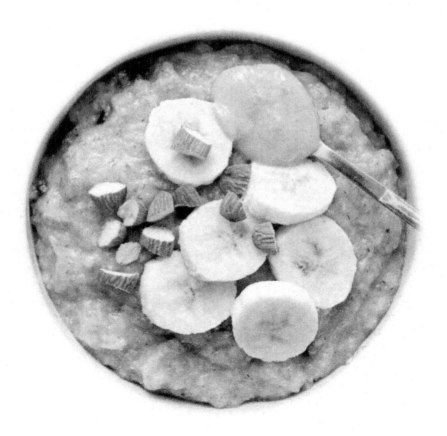

TABLE OF CONTENTS

INTRODUCTION 8

    Importance of Proper Nutrition Post-Surgery...................... 10

CHAPTER ONE 16

    Understanding Gastric Bypass Surgery 16

    Tips for Navigating Food Choices and Portion Control After Surgery 19

CHAPTER TWO 24

Liquid and Pureed Foods Stage Recipes.............................. 24

    Breakfast Recipes.. 24

        Protein-Packed Breakfast Smoothie 24

        Creamy Pumpkin Spice Smoothie 26

        Creamy Vanilla Protein Pudding.................................... 28

        Creamy Avocado and Spinach Smoothie 30

        Banana-Berry Breakfast Bowl 32

        Creamy Peanut Butter Protein Shake............................. 34

        Creamy Strawberry-Banana Protein Smoothie Bowl 36

        Creamy Vanilla Yogurt Parfait 38

        Creamy Blueberry Protein Smoothie 40

        Creamy Vanilla Chia Pudding.. 42

    Lunch Recipes... 44

        Creamy Vegetable Soup... 44

        Creamy Chicken and Spinach Puree.............................. 46

        Creamy Butternut Squash Soup..................................... 48

Creamy Tomato Basil Soup 50

Creamy Broccoli and Cheese Soup.................. 52

Creamy Spinach and Mushroom Puree.................. 54

Creamy Cauliflower and Leek Soup.................. 56

Creamy Asparagus and Potato Puree 58

Creamy Red Lentil Soup.................. 60

Creamy Mushroom and Potato Soup 63

Dinner Recipes.................. 66

Creamy Turkey and Vegetable Puree 66

Creamy Salmon and Cauliflower Mash.................. 68

Creamy Chicken and Mushroom Puree 70

Creamy Lentil and Vegetable Puree.................. 72

Creamy Vegetable and Quinoa Puree 74

Creamy Spinach and Chickpea Puree 76

Creamy Carrot and Ginger Soup.................. 78

Creamy Cauliflower and Spinach Soup.................. 81

Creamy Tomato and Basil Soup.................. 84

Creamy Zucchini and Avocado Soup.................. 87

CHAPTER THREE 90

Soft Foods Stage Recipes.................. 90

Breakfast Recipes.................. 90

Scrambled Eggs with Avocado 90

Greek Yogurt Parfait 92

Cottage Cheese Pancakes.................. 94

Soft Scrambled Tofu 96

Banana Oatmeal Pancakes 98

Soft Scrambled Eggs with Cheese 100

Apple Cinnamon Oatmeal.. 102

Soft Boiled Eggs with Toast Soldiers 104

Creamy Peanut Butter Banana Smoothie........................... 106

Soft Scrambled Tofu Breakfast Bowl 108

Lunch Recipes...110

Turkey and Avocado Wrap..110

Salmon Salad 112

Chicken and Avocado Salad..114

Tuna Salad Lettuce Wraps 116

Egg Salad Lettuce Wraps 118

Quinoa and Vegetable Salad 120

Avocado Tuna Salad 122

Turkey and Hummus Wrap 124

Chicken and Quinoa Bowl.. 126

Shrimp and Avocado Salad 128

Dinner Recipes... 130

Baked Salmon with Mashed Sweet Potatoes 130

Turkey Meatballs with Zucchini Noodles........................... 132

Baked Chicken Breast with Roasted Vegetables................. 135

Lentil Soup... 138

Baked Cod with Roasted Vegetables 140

Turkey Chili 143

Turkey and Vegetable Stir-Fry 146

Vegetable Frittata 149

Lemon Herb Baked Tilapia.................................... 152

Eggplant Parmesan... 154

CHAPTER FOUR.. 158

Regular Foods Stage Recipes... 158

Breakfast Recipes... 158

Veggie Omelette... 158

Greek Yogurt Parfait 161

Avocado Toast with Poached Egg..................... 163

Turkey and Cheese Breakfast Wrap.................. 166

Spinach and Feta Frittata 169

Breakfast Burrito... 172

Smoked Salmon Bagel.. 174

Veggie Breakfast Burrito Bowl.......................... 176

Quinoa Breakfast Bowl....................................... 178

Banana Nut Oatmeal 180

Lunch Recipes... 182

Grilled Chicken Salad... 182

Turkey and Avocado Wrap.................................. 185

Salmon Quinoa Bowl.. 187

Turkey and Vegetable Stir-Fry 190

Quinoa and Black Bean Salad............................ 193

Greek Chicken Pita Pockets............................... 196

Turkey and Veggie Stir-Fry................................. 199

Caprese Chicken Salad 202

Turkey and Quinoa Stuffed Bell Peppers 204

Chicken Caesar Salad 207

Dinner Recipes 210

Baked Lemon Herb Salmon 210

Grilled Chicken and Vegetable Skewers 212

Beef and Vegetable Stir-Fry 214

Shrimp and Asparagus Pasta 217

Baked Chicken Parmesan 220

Turkey and Quinoa Stuffed Bell Peppers 223

Baked Garlic Butter Salmon with Asparagus 226

Turkey Taco Lettuce Wraps 229

Grilled Lemon Herb Chicken Breast 232

Baked Turkey and Vegetable Casserole 234

CHAPTER FIVE 238

Meal Planning and Portion Control 238

Strategies for Planning Meals and Snacks 238

Portion Control Guidelines and Visual Aids 240

CONCLUSION 242

GASTRIC BYPASS COOKBOOK FOR ALL STAGES

INTRODUCTION

Gastric bypass surgery, commonly known as Roux-en-Y gastric bypass (RYGB), is a surgical treatment that aims to assist people with extreme obesity lose weight and improve their health.

This operation includes generating a tiny pouch from the stomach and attaching it straight to the small intestine, skipping a section of the stomach and intestine. This modifies how food is digested and absorbed, resulting in lower calorie intake and, eventually, weight reduction.

The gastric bypass surgery process is separated into numerous stages, each carefully intended to assist patients to gradually adjust to their new eating habits and lifestyle modifications. These steps are critical for ensuring adequate healing, reducing problems, and improving weight reduction results.

Let's delve into each stage to understand its purpose and dietary requirements:

Preoperative Preparation:

Before undergoing gastric bypass surgery, patients are usually evaluated by a multidisciplinary team that includes a surgeon, dietician, psychologist, and other healthcare specialists.

This step includes preoperative counseling, medical exams, and operation preparation. Patients may be needed to follow a preoperative diet to shrink the liver and lower surgery risks.

Immediate Postoperative Stage:

Following surgery, patients enter the immediate postoperative stage, which is characterized by strict monitoring and a gradual return to oral intake.

During this period, patients are usually on a clear liquid diet for the first several days, then advance to a complete liquid diet as tolerated.

This stage allows the surgical site to recover and helps patients become used to drinking tiny amounts of liquids.

Liquid and Pureed Foods Stage:

After successfully tolerating liquids, patients advance to the liquid and pureed meals stage. This stage usually lasts a few weeks and involves eating meals that have been pureed or mixed to a smooth consistency.

Examples include protein smoothies, soups, yogurt, and baby food. The emphasis is on high-protein, low-calorie diets that promote healing and satisfaction.

Soft Foods Stage:

As patients recuperate, they go to the soft foods stage, in which they can gradually incorporate soft, readily digested meals into their diet.

This period allows for a larger variety and texture in meals, such as mashed vegetables, tender meats, eggs, and soft fruit. It is critical to maintain focusing on protein-rich foods while avoiding those high in sugar, fat, or empty calories.

Regular Foods Stage:

The final step of recuperation is the return to regular solid meals, which usually takes many months following surgery. Patients can gradually add a broader range of foods to their diet, such as lean proteins, whole grains, fruits, vegetables, and healthy fats.

However, quantity management is still crucial because the stomach pouch is substantially smaller after surgery, and overeating can cause pain or problems.

Each stage of the gastric bypass surgery journey provides patients with distinct difficulties and opportunity to learn and adjust to their new eating habits and lifestyle.

Patients must collaborate closely with their healthcare team, which includes surgeons, nutritionists, and other experts, to ensure they receive the necessary support and direction for long-term success.

Importance of Proper Nutrition Post-Surgery

Proper nutrition plays a pivotal role in the success of gastric bypass surgery and the overall health and well-being of individuals undergoing this transformative procedure.

The changes made to the digestive system during gastric bypass surgery require careful attention to dietary habits to ensure optimal healing, weight loss, and long-term success.

The importance of proper nutrition post-surgery and how it contributes to the overall success of the procedure include:

Facilitating Healing and Recovery:

Following gastric bypass surgery, the body undergoes significant physiological changes as it adapts to the altered digestive system.

Proper nutrition is essential during this period to support the healing process, promote tissue repair, and reduce the risk of complications.

Adequate intake of protein, vitamins, minerals, and other essential nutrients is crucial for wound healing, immune function, and overall recovery.

Promoting Weight Loss and Management:

One of the primary goals of gastric bypass surgery is to achieve significant and sustainable weight loss. Proper nutrition post-surgery is fundamental to achieving and maintaining this goal. The surgery restricts the size of the stomach pouch and alters the way food is digested and absorbed, leading to reduced calorie intake and weight loss. By focusing on nutrient-dense, low-calorie foods, patients can maximize weight loss outcomes while ensuring they meet their nutritional needs.

Preventing Nutritional Deficiencies:

The altered anatomy and reduced food intake following gastric bypass surgery increase the risk of nutritional deficiencies. Key nutrients such as protein, iron, calcium, vitamin B12, vitamin D, and folate may be inadequately absorbed or consumed in insufficient quantities. It is essential for patients to adhere to a nutrient-rich diet and take prescribed supplements to prevent deficiencies and maintain optimal health.

Supporting Metabolic Health:

Gastric bypass surgery has profound effects on metabolic health, including improvements in insulin sensitivity, blood sugar control, and lipid profiles.

Proper nutrition post-surgery can further enhance these metabolic benefits by promoting stable blood sugar levels, reducing inflammation, and supporting healthy cholesterol levels.

Emphasizing whole, unprocessed foods, lean proteins, and complex carbohydrates can help regulate metabolism and promote overall metabolic health.

Preventing Complications and Long-Term Health Risks:

In addition to supporting weight loss and metabolic health, proper nutrition post-surgery is crucial for preventing complications and reducing the risk of long-term health problems. Obesity-related comorbidities such as type 2 diabetes, hypertension, heart disease, and sleep apnea can be significantly improved or even resolved with successful weight loss and lifestyle modifications. By adopting a nutritious diet and making healthy lifestyle choices, patients can mitigate these risks and enjoy improved overall health and quality of life.

Promoting Long-Term Success and Sustainability:

Sustainable weight loss and long-term success after gastric bypass surgery necessitate a consistent commitment to healthy eating habits and lifestyle adjustments.

Proper nutrition is critical in this process because it provides the essential nutrients required to maintain physical health, mental well-being, and general vigor. Patients can create long-term healthy behaviors by developing a good relationship with food, practicing mindful eating, and making educated food choices.

The goal of this cookbook is to provide a complete resource for those following gastric bypass surgery at all phases of their recovery. Whether you're preparing for surgery, in the early stages of recuperation, or far into your weight loss and lifestyle makeover, this cookbook is here to help you every step of the way.

Our goal is to provide a varied range of appetizing meals that are not only delicious and enjoyable, but also adhere to the strict dietary rules and nutritional requirements related with gastric bypass surgery. Each dish was carefully designed to prioritize protein, vitamins, minerals, and other necessary components while limiting empty calories, sweets, and bad fats.

Furthermore, this cookbook is a useful resource for managing the obstacles and possibilities that come with post-surgery dietary modifications. From meal planning and portion management to eating out and navigating social settings, we offer advice, methods, and insights to help you make educated decisions and live a healthy, balanced lifestyle.

This cookbook is aimed toward those who have had gastric bypass surgery or are considering it as a treatment option for extreme obesity and accompanying health issues. Whether you're looking for ideas for nutritious and tasty dishes, advice on post-surgery nutritional progression, or help adopting healthier eating habits, this cookbook has you covered.

This cookbook is also an excellent resource for healthcare professionals, such as surgeons, dietitians, nurses, and other members of the healthcare team, who work closely with patients following gastric bypass surgery. It offers evidence-based information, practical recommendations, and culinary inspiration to help them promote optimal nutrition, weight control, and general health for their patients.

This cookbook is more than simply a collection of recipes; it is a guide for your road to improved health and a brighter future. By eating healthy, tasty meals and making conscious choices, you may achieve long-term weight loss, better health outcomes, and a higher quality of life.

I welcome you to peruse the pages of this cookbook, try new flavors and ingredients, and find the delight of nourishing your body and spirit on the road to wellbeing.

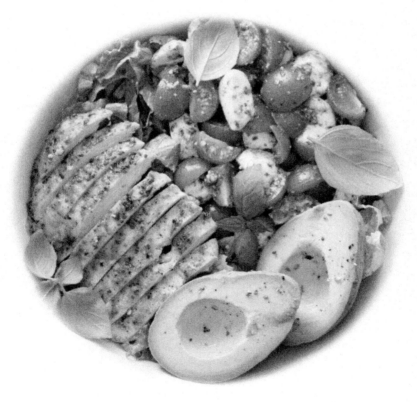

GASTRIC BYPASS COOKBOOK FOR ALL STAGES

CHAPTER ONE
Understanding Gastric Bypass Surgery

Gastric bypass surgery, also known as Roux-en-Y gastric bypass (RYGB), is a life-changing procedure designed to help individuals struggling with severe obesity achieve significant weight loss and improve their overall health.

Central to the success of gastric bypass surgery is the careful management of the different stages of recovery and dietary progression.

Here, we will explore each stage in detail, from the immediate postoperative period to long-term dietary habits which are:

Preoperative Preparation:

Before undergoing gastric bypass surgery, patients must go through a thorough preoperative screening to determine their suitability for the treatment and identify any potential risks or consequences.

This step often includes discussions with a multidisciplinary team that includes a surgeon, dietician, psychologist, and other healthcare specialists. Patients are educated about the procedure, its possible advantages and hazards, and the lifestyle adjustments necessary for long-term success.

In some situations, patients may be instructed to eat a preoperative diet to shrink the liver and lower the chance of surgical problems.

Immediate Postoperative Stage:

The immediate postoperative period begins right after surgery and lasts for the first few days as patients recuperate in the hospital. During this period, healthcare staff constantly check patients' safety and comfort.

The major focus is on pain control, wound care, and a gradual return to oral intake. Initially, patients are put on a clear liquid diet to avoid dehydration and reduce stress on the newly formed stomach pouch.

As tolerated, patients move to sips of water, broth, and sugar-free clear liquids, then to full liquids such protein shakes, yogurt, and diluted fruit juices.

Liquid and Pureed Foods Stage:

Once patients have successfully tolerated liquids and the surgical site has begun to heal, they move on to the liquid and pureed foods stage.

This stage usually lasts a few weeks and involves eating meals that have been pureed or mixed to a smooth consistency. During this period, the major objective is to give enough nourishment while progressively introducing solid meals into the stomach pouch. Protein drinks, creamy soups, smooth yogurt, pureed veggies, and soft fruits are all good options.

Patients are recommended to eat protein-rich meals to aid healing and satiety, while avoiding high-calorie, high-sugar drinks that may inhibit weight reduction.

Soft Foods Stage:

As patients recuperate, they go to the soft foods stage, in which they can gradually incorporate soft, readily digested meals into their diet.

This stage usually comes several weeks following surgery, when the surgical site has healed and patients can handle pureed diets effectively.

Soft meals are simpler to chew and digest than solid foods, making them ideal for people who have a smaller stomach pouch and a different digestive system.

Soft foods include tender meats, fish, poultry, scrambled eggs, cottage cheese, cooked vegetables, and ripe fruit. Patients should chew their meal completely and consume slowly to avoid pain and improve digestion.

Regular Foods Stage:

The final stage of recovery is the return to regular solid meals, which usually takes many months following surgery. By this point, patients have adjusted to their new eating habits and lifestyle changes, and their stomach pouch has recovered enough to handle a broader range of foods.

However, portion management is still crucial since the stomach pouch is substantially smaller after surgery, and overeating can cause pain, vomiting, or pouch straining. Patients are recommended to eat nutrient-dense, high-protein meals such lean meats, fish, poultry, tofu, legumes, whole grains, fruits, and vegetables, while avoiding empty calories, sweets, and harmful fats.

Understanding the various stages of recovery and dietary progression is critical for gastric bypass surgery patients seeking best results and long-term success.

Each stage brings distinct difficulties and chances for patients to learn and adjust to their new eating habits and lifestyle modifications. Patients who comprehend the Gastric Bypass

Surgery may confidently manage their postoperative path and achieve their weight reduction and health goals.

.

Tips for Navigating Food Choices and Portion Control After Surgery

Navigating food choices and portion control after gastric bypass surgery is a critical aspect of achieving long-term success and maintaining a healthy lifestyle.

The surgery alters the anatomy of the digestive system, limiting the amount of food that can be consumed and altering the way nutrients are absorbed. As such, patients must develop new eating habits and strategies to support their weight loss goals and overall well-being.

Here, we will explore various tips and techniques to help patients make informed food choices and practice portion control after surgery which are:

Focus on Nutrient-Dense Foods:

Following gastric bypass surgery, every mouthful matters, therefore select nutrient-dense meals that contain the highest vitamin, mineral, and other critical nutritional value.

Lean proteins like chicken, turkey, fish, eggs, tofu, and lentils should be a staple of your diet since they promote satiety, muscle health, and weight loss. To ensure you're getting enough nutrients, eat a range of colorful fruits and veggies, whole grains, and healthy fats like nuts, seeds, avocado, and olive oil.

Avoid Empty Calories and Sugary Foods:

While it may be tempting to indulge in sweets and high-calorie snacks, these foods are low in nutritious value and might impede weight loss attempts.

After surgery, your stomach pouch shrinks, giving you less capacity for empty calories. Avoid sugary meals, drinks, and processed snacks since they can cause fast blood sugar rises and falls, increase cravings, and contribute to weight gain. Instead, choose naturally sweet fruits, sugar-free options, and sweets in moderation.

Practice Mindful Eating:

Mindful eating is listening to your body's hunger and fullness cues, appreciating each meal, and eating with purpose and awareness.

To avoid overeating and pain after surgery, you should slow down, chew your meal completely, and pay attention to your body's cues. Focus on the flavors, textures, and fragrances of your meals, and stop eating when you're full, not stuffed.

Eating mindfully can help you create a healthy connection with food and make more deliberate decisions about what and how much you consume.

Portion Control Guidelines:

Portion control is key to preventing overeating and promoting weight loss after gastric bypass surgery. Your healthcare team will provide guidance on appropriate portion sizes for each stage of your recovery, but here are some general guidelines to keep in mind:

- Use smaller plates, bowls, and utensils to visually trick your brain into thinking you're eating more.

- Measure or weigh your food portions until you become familiar with appropriate serving sizes.
- Aim to fill half of your plate with non-starchy vegetables, one-quarter with lean protein, and one-quarter with whole grains or starchy vegetables.
- Eat slowly and take breaks between bites to gauge your hunger and fullness levels.

Stay Hydrated:

Adequate hydration is critical to general health and well-being, particularly after gastric bypass surgery. Drink water throughout the day to avoid dehydration, boost satiety, and improve digestion.

Avoid drinking liquids with meals since they can fill up your stomach pouch and keep you from eating enough nutrient-dense foods.

Instead, hydrate between meals and wait at least 30 minutes before and after eating to consume liquids. To increase the diversity of your fluid consumption, try low-calorie, sugar-free liquids like herbal tea, infused water, or broth.

Plan and Prepare Meals in Advance:

Planning and preparing meals ahead of time will help you stick to your dietary objectives and avoid making impulsive food decisions.

Set aside time each week to plan your meals, make a grocery list, and prepare items ahead of time. Cook and divide out meals and snacks for the week ahead of time, making it easy to select healthy alternatives when you're hungry.

Make healthy eating more accessible and simpler by stocking your kitchen with nutritional essentials like pre-cut veggies, prepared meats, and portion-controlled snacks.

Seek Support and Accountability:

Beginning a post-surgical nutritional path might be difficult, but you don't have to do it alone. Seek assistance from friends, family members, and other patients who understand your situation and can provide encouragement, guidance, and inspiration.

Consider joining a support group, attending nutrition counseling sessions, or consulting with a certified dietitian who specializes in bariatric nutrition to help you stay accountable and on track with your objectives.

Navigating food choices and quantity management after gastric bypass surgery needs dedication, patience, and a desire to embrace a new way of eating.

Patients can improve their weight reduction results, nutritional status, and general quality of life by concentrating on nutrient-dense meals, practicing mindful eating, and prioritizing portion management.

By applying these strategies and practices, patients may empower themselves to make educated decisions and develop a long-term, healthy eating plan that supports their success and well-being.

GASTRIC BYPASS COOKBOOK FOR ALL STAGES

CHAPTER TWO
Liquid and Pureed Foods Stage Recipes
Breakfast Recipes

Protein-Packed Breakfast Smoothie

Prep Time: 5 minutes | Cooking Time: 0 minutes | Servings: 1

Ingredients:
- 1/2 cup unsweetened almond milk
- 1/2 cup Greek yogurt (plain or flavored)
- 1 scoop protein powder (vanilla or flavor of choice)
- 1/2 ripe banana, frozen
- 1/4 cup frozen berries (such as strawberries, blueberries, or raspberries)
- 1 tablespoon almond butter or peanut butter (optional)
- 1/2 teaspoon honey or maple syrup (optional, for sweetness)

Method of Preparation:
1. In a blender, combine almond milk, Greek yogurt, protein powder, frozen banana, frozen berries, almond butter (if using), and honey or maple syrup (if using).
2. Blend on high speed until smooth and creamy, scraping down the sides of the blender if necessary.
3. Pour the smoothie into a glass and enjoy immediately.

> *Nutritional Info:*
> *Calories: 300 | Protein: 30g | Carbohydrates: 30g | Fat: 8g | Fiber: 5g*

GASTRIC BYPASS COOKBOOK FOR ALL STAGES

Recipe Name:_____

Date: / /   *Time:_____*

Rating: ☆ ☆ ☆ ☆ ☆

S/N	Ingredients	Adjustment

Cooking Experience: _____

_____

_____

_____

Notes:_____

_____

_____

_____

_____

_____

_____

Creamy Pumpkin Spice Smoothie

Prep Time: 5 minutes | Cooking Time: 0 minutes | Servings: 1

Ingredients:

- 1/2 cup unsweetened almond milk
- 1/2 cup canned pumpkin puree
- 1/2 cup Greek yogurt (plain or vanilla)
- 1 scoop protein powder (vanilla or flavor of choice)
- 1/2 teaspoon ground cinnamon
- 1/4 teaspoon ground nutmeg
- 1/4 teaspoon ground ginger
- 1 tablespoon honey or maple syrup (optional, for sweetness)

Method of Preparation:

1. In a blender, combine almond milk, pumpkin puree, Greek yogurt, protein powder, ground cinnamon, ground nutmeg, ground ginger, and honey or maple syrup (if using).
2. Blend on high speed until smooth and creamy, adjusting sweetness to taste if necessary.
3. Pour the smoothie into a glass and sprinkle with additional ground cinnamon for garnish, if desired. Serve immediately.

Nutritional Info:
Calories: 250 | Protein: 25g | Carbohydrates: 30g | Fat: 5g |
Fiber: 8g

GASTRIC BYPASS COOKBOOK FOR ALL STAGES

Recipe Name:_____

Date: / /   *Time:*_____

Rating: ☆ ☆ ☆ ☆ ☆

S/N	Ingredients	Adjustment

Cooking Experience: _____
_____
_____
_____

Notes:_____
_____
_____
_____
_____
_____
_____

Creamy Vanilla Protein Pudding

Prep Time: 5 minutes | Cooking Time: 0 minutes | Servings: 1

Ingredients:

- 1/2 cup unsweetened almond milk
- 1 scoop vanilla protein powder
- 2 tablespoons chia seeds
- 1/4 teaspoon vanilla extract
- Stevia or monk fruit sweetener, to taste (optional)

Method of Preparation:

1. In a small bowl, whisk together almond milk, vanilla protein powder, chia seeds, vanilla extract, and sweetener (if using) until well combined.
2. Let the mixture sit for 5 minutes to allow the chia seeds to thicken and absorb the liquid.
3. Stir the pudding again, then transfer it to a serving dish. Refrigerate for at least 30 minutes or until chilled and set.
4. Serve the pudding cold, topped with fresh berries or a sprinkle of cinnamon, if desired.

Nutritional Info:
Calories: 250 | Protein: 25g | Carbohydrates: 15g | Fat: 10g | Fiber: 8g

GASTRIC BYPASS COOKBOOK FOR ALL STAGES

Recipe Name:_____

Date: / /   *Time:*_____

Rating: ☆ ☆ ☆ ☆ ☆

S/N	Ingredients	Adjustment

Cooking Experience: _____
_____
_____
_____

Notes:_____
_____
_____
_____
_____
_____
_____

Creamy Avocado and Spinach Smoothie

Prep Time: 5 minutes | Cooking Time: 0 minutes | Servings: 1

Ingredients:

- 1/2 ripe avocado
- 1 cup unsweetened almond milk
- 1 scoop protein powder (unflavored or vanilla)
- 1 handful baby spinach leaves
- 1/2 tablespoon lemon juice
- Stevia or monk fruit sweetener, to taste (optional)

Method of Preparation:

1. In a blender, combine ripe avocado, almond milk, protein powder, baby spinach leaves, lemon juice, and sweetener (if using).
2. Blend on high speed until smooth and creamy, scraping down the sides of the blender if necessary.
3. Pour the smoothie into a glass and serve immediately.

Nutritional Info:
Calories: 300 | Protein: 25g | Carbohydrates: 15g | Fat: 15g | Fiber: 8g

GASTRIC BYPASS COOKBOOK FOR ALL STAGES

Recipe Name:_____

Date: / /   *Time:*_____

Rating: ☆ ☆ ☆ ☆ ☆

S/N	Ingredients	Adjustment

Cooking Experience: _____
_____
_____
_____

Notes:_____
_____
_____
_____
_____
_____
_____

Banana-Berry Breakfast Bowl

Prep Time: 5 minutes | Cooking Time: 0 minutes | Servings: 1

Ingredients:

- 1/2 ripe banana
- 1/2 cup mixed berries (such as strawberries, blueberries, and raspberries)
- 1/4 cup Greek yogurt (plain or flavored)
- 1 tablespoon almond butter or peanut butter
- 1 tablespoon chia seeds
- 1 tablespoon unsweetened coconut flakes (optional)

Method of Preparation:

1. In a small bowl, mash the ripe banana with a fork until smooth.
2. Top the mashed banana with mixed berries, Greek yogurt, almond butter or peanut butter, chia seeds, and unsweetened coconut flakes (if using).
3. Stir to combine all the ingredients, creating a creamy and flavorful breakfast bowl.
4. Enjoy the breakfast bowl immediately, savoring the combination of sweet fruit, creamy yogurt, and nutty flavors.

Nutritional Info:
Calories: 300 | Protein: 15g | Carbohydrates: 30g | Fat: 15g | Fiber: 8g

GASTRIC BYPASS COOKBOOK FOR ALL STAGES

Recipe Name:_____

Date: / /   *Time:*_____

Rating: ☆ ☆ ☆ ☆ ☆

S/N	Ingredients	Adjustment

Cooking Experience: _____
_____
_____
_____

Notes:_____
_____
_____
_____
_____
_____
_____

Creamy Peanut Butter Protein Shake

Prep Time: 5 minutes | Cooking Time: 0 minutes | Servings: 1

Ingredients:

- 1/2 cup unsweetened almond milk
- 1/2 cup Greek yogurt (plain or vanilla)
- 1 scoop protein powder (chocolate or peanut butter flavor)
- 1 tablespoon natural peanut butter
- 1/2 ripe banana, frozen
- 1/4 teaspoon vanilla extract
- Stevia or monk fruit sweetener, to taste (optional)

Method of Preparation:

1. In a blender, combine unsweetened almond milk, Greek yogurt, protein powder, natural peanut butter, frozen banana, vanilla extract, and sweetener (if using).
2. Blend on high speed until smooth and creamy, adjusting sweetness to taste if necessary.
3. Pour the protein shake into a glass and enjoy immediately.

Nutritional Info:
Calories: 350 | Protein: 30g | Carbohydrates: 25g | Fat: 15g |
Fiber: 5g

GASTRIC BYPASS COOKBOOK FOR ALL STAGES

Recipe Name: _____

Date: / /   *Time:*_____

Rating: ☆ ☆ ☆ ☆ ☆

S/N	Ingredients	Adjustment

Cooking Experience: _____

_____
_____
_____

Notes:_____

_____
_____
_____
_____
_____
_____
_____

Creamy Strawberry-Banana Protein Smoothie Bowl

Prep Time: 5 minutes | Cooking Time: 0 minutes | Servings: 1

Ingredients:

- 1/2 ripe banana
- 1/2 cup frozen strawberries
- 1/2 cup Greek yogurt (plain or flavored)
- 1 scoop protein powder (vanilla or strawberry flavor)
- 1 tablespoon almond butter or peanut butter
- 1 tablespoon unsweetened shredded coconut (optional)
- Fresh berries and sliced banana, for topping

Method of Preparation:

1. In a blender, combine the ripe banana, frozen strawberries, Greek yogurt, protein powder, and almond butter or peanut butter.
2. Blend on high speed until smooth and creamy, adding a splash of almond milk if needed to achieve desired consistency.
3. Pour the smoothie into a bowl and sprinkle with unsweetened shredded coconut, if using.
4. Top with fresh berries and sliced banana for added flavor and texture.
5. Enjoy the smoothie bowl immediately with a spoon, savoring the creamy texture and fruity flavors.

> ### Nutritional Info:
> *Calories: 320 | Protein: 25g | Carbohydrates: 30g | Fat: 12g | Fiber: 6g*

GASTRIC BYPASS COOKBOOK FOR ALL STAGES

Recipe Name:_____

Date: / /   *Time:*_____

Rating: ☆ ☆ ☆ ☆ ☆

S/N	Ingredients	Adjustment

Cooking Experience: _____
_____
_____
_____

Notes:_____
_____
_____
_____
_____
_____

Creamy Vanilla Yogurt Parfait

Prep Time: 5 minutes | Cooking Time: 0 minutes | Servings: 1

Ingredients:

- 1/2 cup Greek yogurt (plain or vanilla)
- 1/4 cup unsweetened applesauce
- 1 tablespoon almond butter or peanut butter
- 1 tablespoon chia seeds
- 1/4 teaspoon ground cinnamon
- 1/4 cup fresh berries (such as blueberries or raspberries)

Method of Preparation:

1. In a small bowl, layer Greek yogurt, unsweetened applesauce, almond butter or peanut butter, chia seeds, and ground cinnamon.
2. Repeat the layers until all ingredients are used, creating a visually appealing parfait.
3. Top the parfait with fresh berries for added flavor and nutrition.
4. Serve the yogurt parfait immediately, savoring the creamy texture and delicious combination of flavors.

Nutritional Info:
Calories: 280 | Protein: 20g | Carbohydrates: 25g | Fat: 10g |
Fiber: 8g

GASTRIC BYPASS COOKBOOK FOR ALL STAGES

Recipe Name:_____

Date: / /   *Time:*_____

Rating: ☆ ☆ ☆ ☆ ☆

S/N	Ingredients	Adjustment

Cooking Experience: _____
_____
_____
_____

Notes:_____
_____
_____
_____
_____
_____
_____
_____

Creamy Blueberry Protein Smoothie

Prep Time: 5 minutes | Cooking Time: 0 minutes | Servings: 1

Ingredients:

- 1/2 cup unsweetened almond milk
- 1/2 cup Greek yogurt (plain or blueberry flavored)
- 1 scoop protein powder (vanilla or berry flavor)
- 1/2 cup frozen blueberries
- 1 tablespoon almond butter or cashew butter
- 1 teaspoon honey or maple syrup (optional, for sweetness)
- 1 tablespoon ground flaxseed (optional, for added fiber)

Method of Preparation:

1. In a blender, combine almond milk, Greek yogurt, protein powder, frozen blueberries, almond butter or cashew butter, honey or maple syrup (if using), and ground flaxseed (if using).
2. Blend on high speed until smooth and creamy, adding more almond milk if needed to reach desired consistency.
3. Pour the smoothie into a glass and enjoy immediately, savoring the fruity flavors and creamy texture.

Nutritional Info:
Calories: 320 | Protein: 25g | Carbohydrates: 25g | Fat: 12g | Fiber: 6g

GASTRIC BYPASS COOKBOOK FOR ALL STAGES

Recipe Name:_____

Date: / /   *Time:*_____

Rating: ☆ ☆ ☆ ☆ ☆

S/N	Ingredients	Adjustment

Cooking Experience: _____

_____

_____

_____

Notes:_____

_____

_____

_____

_____

_____

_____

Creamy Vanilla Chia Pudding

Prep Time: 5 minutes | Cooking Time: 0 minutes | Servings: 1

Ingredients:

- 1/2 cup unsweetened almond milk
- 2 tablespoons chia seeds
- 1/2 teaspoon vanilla extract
- Stevia or monk fruit sweetener, to taste (optional)
- Fresh berries or sliced fruit, for topping

Method of Preparation:

1. In a small bowl or glass jar, combine almond milk, chia seeds, vanilla extract, and sweetener (if using).
2. Stir well to combine all ingredients, ensuring the chia seeds are evenly distributed.
3. Cover the bowl or jar and refrigerate for at least 2 hours or overnight to allow the chia seeds to thicken and absorb the liquid.
4. Once the chia pudding has set, stir again to break up any clumps and achieve a smooth consistency.
5. Top the chia pudding with fresh berries or sliced fruit for added flavor and nutrition.
6. Serve the chia pudding cold, enjoying the creamy texture and satisfying taste.

Nutritional Info:
Calories: 200 | Protein: 8g | Carbohydrates: 20g | Fat: 10g | Fiber: 12g

GASTRIC BYPASS COOKBOOK FOR ALL STAGES

Recipe Name:_____

Date: / /   *Time:*_____

Rating: ☆ ☆ ☆ ☆ ☆

S/N	Ingredients	Adjustment

Cooking Experience: _____

_____

_____

_____

Notes:_____

_____

_____

_____

_____

_____

_____

Lunch Recipes

Creamy Vegetable Soup

Prep Time: 10 minutes | Cooking Time: 15 minutes | Servings: 2

Ingredients:

- 1 cup low-sodium vegetable broth
- 1 cup mixed vegetables (such as carrots, celery, and zucchini), chopped
- 1/2 cup cauliflower florets
- 1/4 cup Greek yogurt
- Salt and pepper, to taste
- Fresh herbs (such as parsley or chives), for garnish (optional)

Method of Preparation:

1. In a medium saucepan, bring the vegetable broth to a simmer over medium heat.
2. Add the mixed vegetables and cauliflower florets to the saucepan, and cook until tender, about 10-12 minutes.
3. Once the vegetables are cooked, remove the saucepan from heat and let it cool slightly.
4. Using a blender or immersion blender, puree the cooked vegetables until smooth.
5. Return the pureed soup to the saucepan, and stir in the Greek yogurt until well combined.
6. Season the soup with salt and pepper to taste.
7. Reheat the soup over low heat until warmed through, being careful not to boil.
8. Serve the creamy vegetable soup hot, garnished with fresh herbs if desired.

Nutritional Info:
Calories: 70 | Protein: 5g | Carbohydrates: 10g | Fat: 1g | Fiber: 3g

GASTRIC BYPASS COOKBOOK FOR ALL STAGES

Recipe Name:_____

Date: / /   *Time:_____*

Rating: ☆ ☆ ☆ ☆ ☆

S/N	Ingredients	Adjustment

Cooking Experience: _____
_____
_____
_____

Notes:_____
_____
_____
_____
_____
_____
_____

Creamy Chicken and Spinach Puree

Prep Time: 10 minutes | Cooking Time: 15 minutes | Servings: 2

Ingredients:

- 1 cup cooked chicken breast, shredded
- 1 cup low-sodium chicken broth
- 1 cup fresh spinach leaves
- 1/4 cup Greek yogurt
- Salt and pepper, to taste

Method of Preparation:

1. In a medium saucepan, combine the cooked chicken breast and chicken broth.
2. Bring the mixture to a simmer over medium heat, and cook for 5 minutes to warm the chicken.
3. Add the fresh spinach leaves to the saucepan, and cook for an additional 2-3 minutes until wilted.
4. Remove the saucepan from heat, and let it cool slightly.
5. Using a blender or immersion blender, puree the chicken and spinach mixture until smooth.
6. Return the pureed mixture to the saucepan, and stir in the Greek yogurt until well combined.
7. Season the puree with salt and pepper to taste.
8. Reheat the puree over low heat until warmed through, stirring occasionally.
9. Serve the creamy chicken and spinach puree hot, garnished with a sprinkle of black pepper if desired.

Nutritional Info:
Calories: 120 | Protein: 15g | Carbohydrates: 3g | Fat: 3g | Fiber: 1g

GASTRIC BYPASS COOKBOOK FOR ALL STAGES

Recipe Name:_____

Date: / / *Time:*_____

Rating: ☆ ☆ ☆ ☆ ☆

S/N	Ingredients	Adjustment

Cooking Experience: _____

_____

_____

_____

Notes:_____

_____

_____

_____

_____

_____

_____

_____

Creamy Butternut Squash Soup

Prep Time: 10 minutes | Cooking Time: 25 minutes | Servings: 2

Ingredients:

- 1 cup butternut squash, peeled and diced
- 1/2 cup carrot, peeled and chopped
- 1/4 cup onion, chopped
- 1 cup low-sodium vegetable broth
- 1/4 cup Greek yogurt
- Salt and pepper, to taste
- Fresh parsley, for garnish (optional)

Method of Preparation:

1. In a medium saucepan, combine the diced butternut squash, chopped carrot, chopped onion, and vegetable broth.
2. Bring the mixture to a boil over medium heat, then reduce the heat to low and simmer for 20-25 minutes until the vegetables are tender.
3. Remove the saucepan from heat and let it cool slightly.
4. Using a blender or immersion blender, puree the cooked vegetables and broth until smooth.
5. Return the pureed soup to the saucepan and stir in the Greek yogurt until well combined.
6. Season the soup with salt and pepper to taste.
7. Reheat the soup over low heat until warmed through, being careful not to boil.
8. Serve the creamy butternut squash soup hot, garnished with fresh parsley if desired.

Nutritional Info:
Calories: 90 | Protein: 5g | Carbohydrates: 15g | Fat: 1g | Fiber: 4g

GASTRIC BYPASS COOKBOOK FOR ALL STAGES

Recipe Name:_____

Date: / /   *Time:*_____

Rating: ☆ ☆ ☆ ☆ ☆

S/N	Ingredients	Adjustment

Cooking Experience: _____
_____
_____
_____

Notes:_____
_____
_____
_____
_____
_____
_____
_____

Creamy Tomato Basil Soup

Prep Time: 10 minutes | Cooking Time: 20 minutes | Servings: 2

Ingredients:

- 1 cup canned diced tomatoes
- 1/2 cup low-sodium vegetable broth
- 1/4 cup Greek yogurt
- 1 tablespoon tomato paste
- 2 cloves garlic, minced
- 1/4 teaspoon dried basil
- Salt and pepper, to taste
- Fresh basil leaves, for garnish (optional)

Method of Preparation:

1. In a medium saucepan, combine the canned diced tomatoes, vegetable broth, Greek yogurt, tomato paste, minced garlic, and dried basil.
2. Bring the mixture to a boil over medium heat, then reduce the heat to low and simmer for 15-20 minutes.
3. Remove the saucepan from heat and let it cool slightly.
4. Using a blender or immersion blender, puree the cooked tomato mixture until smooth.
5. Return the pureed soup to the saucepan and season with salt and pepper to taste.
6. Reheat the soup over low heat until warmed through, stirring occasionally.
7. Serve the creamy tomato basil soup hot, garnished with fresh basil leaves if desired.

Nutritional Info:
Calories: 80 | Protein: 5g | Carbohydrates: 15g | Fat: 1g | Fiber: 4g

GASTRIC BYPASS COOKBOOK FOR ALL STAGES

Recipe Name:_____

Date: / /   *Time:*_____

Rating: ☆ ☆ ☆ ☆ ☆

S/N	Ingredients	Adjustment

Cooking Experience: _____
_____
_____
_____

Notes:_____
_____
_____
_____
_____
_____
_____

Creamy Broccoli and Cheese Soup

Prep Time: 10 minutes | Cooking Time: 20 minutes | Servings: 2

Ingredients:

- 1 cup broccoli florets
- 1/2 cup cauliflower florets
- 1/4 cup chopped onion
- 1 cup low-sodium vegetable broth
- 1/4 cup Greek yogurt
- 1/4 cup shredded low-fat cheddar cheese
- Salt and pepper, to taste

Method of Preparation:

1. In a medium saucepan, combine the broccoli florets, cauliflower florets, chopped onion, and vegetable broth.
2. Bring the mixture to a boil over medium heat, then reduce the heat to low and simmer for 15-20 minutes until the vegetables are tender.
3. Remove the saucepan from heat and let it cool slightly.
4. Using a blender or immersion blender, puree the cooked vegetables and broth until smooth.
5. Return the pureed soup to the saucepan and stir in the Greek yogurt until well combined.
6. Add the shredded cheddar cheese to the soup and stir until melted and creamy.
7. Season the soup with salt and pepper to taste.
8. Reheat the soup over low heat until warmed through, stirring occasionally.
9. Serve the creamy broccoli and cheese soup hot, garnished with additional shredded cheese if desired.

Nutritional Info: Calories: 120 | Protein: 10g | Carbohydrates: 15g | Fat: 4g | Fiber: 4g

GASTRIC BYPASS COOKBOOK FOR ALL STAGES

Recipe Name:_____

Date: / /   *Time:*_____

Rating: ☆ ☆ ☆ ☆ ☆

S/N	Ingredients	Adjustment

Cooking Experience: _____
_____
_____
_____

Notes:_____
_____
_____
_____
_____
_____
_____
_____

Creamy Spinach and Mushroom Puree

Prep Time: 10 minutes | Cooking Time: 20 minutes | Servings: 2

Ingredients:

- 1 cup chopped spinach
- 1/2 cup sliced mushrooms
- 1/4 cup chopped onion
- 1 cup low-sodium vegetable broth
- 1/4 cup Greek yogurt
- Salt and pepper, to taste
- Fresh parsley, for garnish (optional)

Method of Preparation:

1. In a medium saucepan, combine the chopped spinach, sliced mushrooms, chopped onion, and vegetable broth.
2. Bring the mixture to a boil over medium heat, then reduce the heat to low and simmer for 15-20 minutes until the vegetables are tender.
3. Remove the saucepan from heat and let it cool slightly.
4. Using a blender or immersion blender, puree the cooked vegetables and broth until smooth.
5. Return the pureed mixture to the saucepan and stir in the Greek yogurt until well combined.
6. Season the puree with salt and pepper to taste.
7. Reheat the puree over low heat until warmed through, stirring occasionally.
8. Serve the creamy spinach and mushroom puree hot, garnished with fresh parsley if desired.

Nutritional Info:
Calories: 100 | Protein: 8g | Carbohydrates: 12g | Fat: 3g | Fiber: 4g

GASTRIC BYPASS COOKBOOK FOR ALL STAGES

Recipe Name:_____

Date: / /   *Time:*_____

Rating: ☆ ☆ ☆ ☆ ☆

S/N	Ingredients	Adjustment

Cooking Experience: _____
_____
_____
_____

Notes:_____
_____
_____
_____
_____
_____
_____

Creamy Cauliflower and Leek Soup

Prep Time: 10 minutes | Cooking Time: 25 minutes | Servings: 2

Ingredients:

- 1 cup cauliflower florets
- 1/2 cup chopped leeks
- 1/4 cup chopped onion
- 1 cup low-sodium vegetable broth
- 1/4 cup Greek yogurt
- 1 tablespoon olive oil
- Salt and pepper, to taste
- Fresh chives, for garnish (optional)

Method of Preparation:

1. In a medium saucepan, heat olive oil over medium heat. Add chopped leeks and onion, and sauté until softened, about 5 minutes.
2. Add cauliflower florets and vegetable broth to the saucepan. Bring to a boil, then reduce heat and simmer until cauliflower is tender, about 15 minutes.
3. Remove the saucepan from heat and let it cool slightly.
4. Using a blender or immersion blender, puree the cooked vegetables and broth until smooth.
5. Return the pureed mixture to the saucepan and stir in the Greek yogurt until well combined.
6. Season the soup with salt and pepper to taste.
7. Reheat the soup over low heat until warmed through, stirring occasionally.
8. Serve the creamy cauliflower and leek soup hot, garnished with fresh chives if desired.

Nutritional Info: Calories: 110 | Protein: 5g | Carbohydrates: 12g | Fat: 5g | Fiber: 4g

GASTRIC BYPASS COOKBOOK FOR ALL STAGES

Recipe Name:_____

Date: / /   *Time:*_____

Rating: ☆ ☆ ☆ ☆ ☆

S/N	Ingredients	Adjustment

Cooking Experience: _____
_____
_____
_____

Notes:_____
_____
_____
_____
_____
_____
_____

Creamy Asparagus and Potato Puree

Prep Time: 10 minutes | Cooking Time: 25 minutes | Servings: 2

Ingredients:

- 1 cup chopped asparagus spears
- 1/2 cup diced potato
- 1/4 cup chopped onion
- 1 cup low-sodium vegetable broth
- 1/4 cup Greek yogurt
- 1 tablespoon butter
- Salt and pepper, to taste
- Fresh parsley, for garnish (optional)

Method of Preparation:

1. In a medium saucepan, melt butter over medium heat. Add chopped onion and sauté until softened, about 5 minutes.
2. Add diced potato, chopped asparagus, and vegetable broth to the saucepan. Bring to a boil, then reduce heat and simmer until vegetables are tender, about 15 minutes.
3. Remove the saucepan from heat and let it cool slightly.
4. Using a blender or immersion blender, puree the cooked vegetables and broth until smooth.
5. Return the pureed mixture to the saucepan and stir in the Greek yogurt until well combined.
6. Season the puree with salt and pepper to taste.
7. Reheat the puree over low heat until warmed through, stirring occasionally.
8. Serve the creamy asparagus and potato puree hot, garnished with fresh parsley if desired.

Nutritional Info:
Calories: 120 | Protein: 5g | Carbohydrates: 15g | Fat: 6g | Fiber: 4g

GASTRIC BYPASS COOKBOOK FOR ALL STAGES

Recipe Name:_____

Date: / /   *Time:*_____

Rating: ☆ ☆ ☆ ☆ ☆

S/N	Ingredients	Adjustment

Cooking Experience: _____

_____

_____

_____

Notes:_____

_____

_____

_____

_____

_____

_____

Creamy Red Lentil Soup

Prep Time: 10 minutes | Cooking Time: 25 minutes | Servings: 2

Ingredients:

- 1/2 cup red lentils, rinsed and drained
- 1 cup low-sodium vegetable broth
- 1/2 cup diced carrots
- 1/4 cup diced onion
- 1 clove garlic, minced
- 1/4 teaspoon ground cumin
- 1/4 teaspoon ground turmeric
- 1/4 cup Greek yogurt
- Salt and pepper, to taste
- Fresh cilantro, for garnish (optional)

Method of Preparation:

1. In a medium saucepan, combine red lentils, vegetable broth, diced carrots, diced onion, minced garlic, ground cumin, and ground turmeric.
2. Bring the mixture to a boil over medium heat, then reduce heat to low and simmer for 20-25 minutes until lentils and vegetables are tender.
3. Remove the saucepan from heat and let it cool slightly.
4. Using a blender or immersion blender, puree the cooked lentils and vegetables until smooth.
5. Return the pureed soup to the saucepan and stir in the Greek yogurt until well combined.
6. Season the soup with salt and pepper to taste.
7. Reheat the soup over low heat until warmed through, stirring occasionally.
8. Serve the creamy red lentil soup hot, garnished with fresh cilantro if desired.

Nutritional Info: Calories: 150 | Protein: 10g | Carbohydrates: 25g | Fat: 1g | Fiber: 8g

GASTRIC BYPASS COOKBOOK FOR ALL STAGES

Recipe Name:_____

Date: / /   *Time:*_____

Rating: ☆ ☆ ☆ ☆ ☆

S/N	Ingredients	Adjustment

Cooking Experience: _____

_____
_____
_____

Notes:_____

_____
_____
_____
_____
_____
_____

Creamy Mushroom and Potato Soup

Prep Time: 10 minutes | Cooking Time: 25 minutes | Servings: 2

Ingredients:

- 1 cup sliced mushrooms
- 1/2 cup diced potato
- 1/4 cup chopped onion
- 1 cup low-sodium vegetable broth
- 1/4 cup Greek yogurt
- 1 tablespoon olive oil
- Salt and pepper, to taste
- Fresh thyme, for garnish (optional)

Method of Preparation:

1. In a medium saucepan, heat olive oil over medium heat. Add chopped onion and sauté until softened, about 5 minutes.
2. Add sliced mushrooms and diced potato to the saucepan. Cook for 5-7 minutes until mushrooms are tender.
3. Add vegetable broth to the saucepan and bring to a boil. Reduce heat and simmer for 10-15 minutes until potatoes are cooked through.
4. Remove the saucepan from heat and let it cool slightly.
5. Using a blender or immersion blender, puree the cooked mushrooms, potatoes, and broth until smooth.
6. Return the pureed soup to the saucepan and stir in the Greek yogurt until well combined.
7. Season the soup with salt and pepper to taste.
8. Reheat the soup over low heat until warmed through, stirring occasionally.
9. Serve the creamy mushroom and potato soup hot, garnished with fresh thyme if desired.

> **Nutritional Info:**
> Calories: 140 | Protein: 6g | Carbohydrates: 20g | Fat: 4g | Fiber: 4g

GASTRIC BYPASS COOKBOOK FOR ALL STAGES

Recipe Name:_____

Date: / /   *Time:*_____

Rating: ☆ ☆ ☆ ☆ ☆

S/N	Ingredients	Adjustment

Cooking Experience: _____
_____
_____
_____

Notes:_____
_____
_____
_____
_____
_____
_____

Dinner Recipes

Creamy Turkey and Vegetable Puree

Prep Time: 10 minutes | Cooking Time: 20 minutes | Servings: 2

Ingredients:

- 1/2 cup cooked ground turkey
- 1/2 cup cooked mixed vegetables (such as carrots, peas, and green beans)
- 1/4 cup low-sodium chicken broth
- 1/4 cup Greek yogurt
- Salt and pepper, to taste

Method of Preparation:

1. In a small saucepan, combine cooked ground turkey, cooked mixed vegetables, and low-sodium chicken broth.
2. Heat the mixture over medium heat until warmed through, stirring occasionally.
3. Remove the saucepan from heat and let it cool slightly.
4. Using a blender or immersion blender, puree the cooked turkey, vegetables, and broth until smooth.
5. Return the pureed mixture to the saucepan and stir in the Greek yogurt until well combined.
6. Season the puree with salt and pepper to taste.
7. Reheat the puree over low heat until warmed through, stirring occasionally.
8. Serve the creamy turkey and vegetable puree hot, adjusting seasoning if necessary.

Nutritional Info:
Calories: 150 | Protein: 15g | Carbohydrates: 10g | Fat: 5g | Fiber: 3g

GASTRIC BYPASS COOKBOOK FOR ALL STAGES

Recipe Name:_____

Date: / /   *Time:_____*

Rating: ☆ ☆ ☆ ☆ ☆

S/N	Ingredients	Adjustment

Cooking Experience: _____

_____
_____
_____

Notes:_____

_____
_____
_____
_____
_____
_____
_____

Creamy Salmon and Cauliflower Mash

Prep Time: 10 minutes | Cooking Time: 20 minutes | Servings: 2

Ingredients:

- 1/2 cup cooked salmon, flaked
- 1 cup cooked cauliflower florets
- 1/4 cup low-sodium vegetable broth
- 1/4 cup Greek yogurt
- 1 tablespoon lemon juice
- Salt and pepper, to taste
- Fresh dill, for garnish (optional)

Method of Preparation:

1. In a small saucepan, combine cooked salmon, cooked cauliflower florets, low-sodium vegetable broth, and lemon juice.
2. Heat the mixture over medium heat until warmed through, stirring occasionally.
3. Remove the saucepan from heat and let it cool slightly.
4. Using a blender or immersion blender, puree the cooked salmon, cauliflower, broth, and lemon juice until smooth.
5. Return the pureed mixture to the saucepan and stir in the Greek yogurt until well combined.
6. Season the puree with salt and pepper to taste.
7. Reheat the puree over low heat until warmed through, stirring occasionally.
8. Serve the creamy salmon and cauliflower mash hot, garnished with fresh dill if desired.

Nutritional Info:
Calories: 180 | Protein: 20g | Carbohydrates: 10g | Fat: 7g | Fiber: 4g

GASTRIC BYPASS COOKBOOK FOR ALL STAGES

Recipe Name:_____

Date: / /   *Time:*_____

Rating: ☆ ☆ ☆ ☆ ☆

S/N	Ingredients	Adjustment

Cooking Experience: _____
_____
_____
_____

Notes:_____
_____
_____
_____
_____
_____
_____

Creamy Chicken and Mushroom Puree

Prep Time: 10 minutes | Cooking Time: 20 minutes | Servings: 2

Ingredients:
- 1/2 cup cooked chicken breast, shredded
- 1 cup cooked mushrooms, sliced
- 1/4 cup low-sodium chicken broth
- 1/4 cup Greek yogurt
- 1 tablespoon olive oil
- Salt and pepper, to taste

Method of Preparation:
1. In a small saucepan, heat olive oil over medium heat. Add sliced mushrooms and sauté until softened, about 5 minutes.
2. Add shredded chicken breast and low-sodium chicken broth to the saucepan. Heat the mixture until warmed through, stirring occasionally.
3. Remove the saucepan from heat and let it cool slightly.
4. Using a blender or immersion blender, puree the cooked chicken, mushrooms, and broth until smooth.
5. Return the pureed mixture to the saucepan and stir in the Greek yogurt until well combined.
6. Season the puree with salt and pepper to taste.
7. Reheat the puree over low heat until warmed through, stirring occasionally.
8. Serve the creamy chicken and mushroom puree hot, adjusting seasoning if necessary.

Nutritional Info:
Calories: 160 | Protein: 15g | Carbohydrates: 8g | Fat: 7g | Fiber: 2g

Recipe Name:_____

Date: / /   *Time:*_____

Rating: ☆ ☆ ☆ ☆ ☆

S/N	Ingredients	Adjustment

Cooking Experience: _____

_____

_____

_____

Notes:_____

_____

_____

_____

_____

_____

_____

Creamy Lentil and Vegetable Puree

Prep Time: 10 minutes | Cooking Time: 25 minutes | Servings: 2

Ingredients:

- 1/2 cup cooked lentils
- 1/2 cup cooked mixed vegetables (such as carrots, peas, and corn)
- 1/4 cup low-sodium vegetable broth
- 1/4 cup Greek yogurt
- 1 tablespoon olive oil
- Salt and pepper, to taste

Method of Preparation:

1. In a small saucepan, heat olive oil over medium heat. Add cooked lentils and mixed vegetables to the saucepan. Heat the mixture until warmed through, stirring occasionally.
2. Add low-sodium vegetable broth to the saucepan and simmer for 5-7 minutes until flavors meld.
3. Remove the saucepan from heat and let it cool slightly.
4. Using a blender or immersion blender, puree the cooked lentils, vegetables, and broth until smooth.
5. Return the pureed mixture to the saucepan and stir in the Greek yogurt until well combined.
6. Season the puree with salt and pepper to taste.
7. Reheat the puree over low heat until warmed through, stirring occasionally.
8. Serve the creamy lentil and vegetable puree hot, adjusting seasoning if necessary.

Nutritional Info:
Calories: 150 | Protein: 10g | Carbohydrates: 20g | Fat: 5g | Fiber: 6g

GASTRIC BYPASS COOKBOOK FOR ALL STAGES

Recipe Name:_____

Date: / /   *Time:*_____

Rating: ☆ ☆ ☆ ☆ ☆

S/N	Ingredients	Adjustment

Cooking Experience: _____
_____
_____
_____

Notes:_____
_____
_____
_____
_____
_____
_____

Creamy Vegetable and Quinoa Puree

Prep Time: 10 minutes | Cooking Time: 25 minutes | Servings: 2

Ingredients:

- 1/2 cup cooked quinoa
- 1 cup cooked mixed vegetables (such as carrots, broccoli, and cauliflower)
- 1/4 cup low-sodium vegetable broth
- 1/4 cup Greek yogurt
- Salt and pepper, to taste

Method of Preparation:

1. In a small saucepan, combine cooked quinoa, mixed vegetables, and low-sodium vegetable broth.
2. Heat the mixture over medium heat until warmed through, stirring occasionally.
3. Remove the saucepan from heat and let it cool slightly.
4. Using a blender or immersion blender, puree the cooked quinoa, vegetables, and broth until smooth.
5. Return the pureed mixture to the saucepan and stir in the Greek yogurt until well combined.
6. Season the puree with salt and pepper to taste.
7. Reheat the puree over low heat until warmed through, stirring occasionally.
8. Serve the creamy vegetable and quinoa puree hot, adjusting seasoning if necessary.

Nutritional Info:
Calories: 160 | Protein: 8g | Carbohydrates: 25g | Fat: 3g | Fiber: 5g

GASTRIC BYPASS COOKBOOK FOR ALL STAGES

Recipe Name:_____

Date: / /   *Time:*_____

Rating: ☆ ☆ ☆ ☆ ☆

S/N	Ingredients	Adjustment

Cooking Experience: _____
_____
_____
_____

Notes:_____
_____
_____
_____
_____
_____
_____

Creamy Spinach and Chickpea Puree

Prep Time: 10 minutes | Cooking Time: 20 minutes | Servings: 2

Ingredients:

- 1 cup cooked chickpeas
- 1 cup chopped spinach
- 1/4 cup low-sodium vegetable broth
- 1/4 cup Greek yogurt
- 1 tablespoon olive oil
- Salt and pepper, to taste

Method of Preparation:

1. In a small saucepan, heat olive oil over medium heat. Add chopped spinach and sauté until wilted, about 3-5 minutes.
2. Add cooked chickpeas and low-sodium vegetable broth to the saucepan. Heat the mixture until warmed through, stirring occasionally.
3. Remove the saucepan from heat and let it cool slightly.
4. Using a blender or immersion blender, puree the cooked chickpeas, spinach, and broth until smooth.
5. Return the pureed mixture to the saucepan and stir in the Greek yogurt until well combined.
6. Season the puree with salt and pepper to taste.
7. Reheat the puree over low heat until warmed through, stirring occasionally.
8. Serve the creamy spinach and chickpea puree hot, adjusting seasoning if necessary.

Nutritional Info:
Calories: 180 | Protein: 9g | Carbohydrates: 22g | Fat: 6g | Fiber: 7g

GASTRIC BYPASS COOKBOOK FOR ALL STAGES

Recipe Name:_____

Date: / /   *Time:_____*

Rating: ☆ ☆ ☆ ☆ ☆

S/N	Ingredients	Adjustment

Cooking Experience: _____

_____

_____

_____

Notes:_____

_____

_____

_____

_____

_____

_____

Creamy Carrot and Ginger Soup

Prep Time: 10 minutes | Cooking Time: 25 minutes | Servings: 2

Ingredients:

- 1 cup chopped carrots
- 1/4 cup chopped onion
- 1 teaspoon grated ginger
- 1 cup low-sodium vegetable broth
- 1/4 cup Greek yogurt
- 1 tablespoon olive oil
- Salt and pepper, to taste
- Fresh cilantro, for garnish (optional)

Method of Preparation:

1. In a medium saucepan, heat olive oil over medium heat. Add chopped carrots and onion, and sauté until softened, about 5 minutes.
2. Add grated ginger to the saucepan and cook for another 2 minutes until fragrant.
3. Pour in the low-sodium vegetable broth and bring to a boil. Reduce heat to low and simmer for 15-20 minutes until carrots are tender.
4. Remove the saucepan from heat and let it cool slightly.
5. Using a blender or immersion blender, puree the cooked carrots, onion, ginger, and broth until smooth.
6. Return the pureed mixture to the saucepan and stir in the Greek yogurt until well combined.
7. Season the soup with salt and pepper to taste.
8. Reheat the soup over low heat until warmed through, stirring occasionally.
9. Serve the creamy carrot and ginger soup hot, garnished with fresh cilantro if desired.

> **Nutritional Info:**
> Calories: 120 | Protein: 4g | Carbohydrates: 18g | Fat: 5g | Fiber: 4g

GASTRIC BYPASS COOKBOOK FOR ALL STAGES

Recipe Name:_____

Date: / /   *Time:*_____

Rating: ☆ ☆ ☆ ☆ ☆

S/N	Ingredients	Adjustment

Cooking Experience: _____

_____

_____

_____

Notes:_____

_____

_____

_____

_____

_____

_____

Creamy Cauliflower and Spinach Soup

Prep Time: 10 minutes | Cooking Time: 25 minutes | Servings: 2

Ingredients:

- 1 cup chopped cauliflower
- 1 cup chopped spinach
- 1/4 cup chopped onion
- 1 clove garlic, minced
- 1 cup low-sodium vegetable broth
- 1/4 cup Greek yogurt
- 1 tablespoon olive oil
- Salt and pepper, to taste
- Fresh parsley, for garnish (optional)

Method of Preparation:

1. In a medium saucepan, heat olive oil over medium heat. Add chopped onion and garlic, and sauté until softened, about 5 minutes.
2. Add chopped cauliflower and vegetable broth to the saucepan. Bring to a boil, then reduce heat and simmer for 15-20 minutes until cauliflower is tender.
3. Stir in chopped spinach and cook for an additional 2-3 minutes until wilted.
4. Remove the saucepan from heat and let it cool slightly.
5. Using a blender or immersion blender, puree the cooked cauliflower, spinach, onion, garlic, and broth until smooth.
6. Return the pureed mixture to the saucepan and stir in the Greek yogurt until well combined.
7. Season the soup with salt and pepper to taste.
8. Reheat the soup over low heat until warmed through, stirring occasionally.

9. Serve the creamy cauliflower and spinach soup hot, garnished with fresh parsley if desired.

Nutritional Info:
Calories: 110 | Protein: 5g | Carbohydrates: 15g | Fat: 5g | Fiber: 5g

GASTRIC BYPASS COOKBOOK FOR ALL STAGES

Recipe Name:_____

Date: / /   *Time:*_____

Rating: ☆ ☆ ☆ ☆ ☆

S/N	Ingredients	Adjustment

Cooking Experience: _____
_____
_____
_____

Notes:_____
_____
_____
_____
_____
_____
_____

Creamy Tomato and Basil Soup

Prep Time: 10 minutes | Cooking Time: 25 minutes | Servings: 2

Ingredients:

- 1 cup chopped tomatoes
- 1/4 cup chopped onion
- 1 clove garlic, minced
- 1 tablespoon tomato paste
- 1 cup low-sodium vegetable broth
- 1/4 cup Greek yogurt
- 1 tablespoon olive oil
- Salt and pepper, to taste
- Fresh basil leaves, for garnish (optional)

Method of Preparation:

1. In a medium saucepan, heat olive oil over medium heat. Add chopped onion and garlic, and sauté until softened, about 5 minutes.
2. Add chopped tomatoes and tomato paste to the saucepan. Cook for another 5 minutes until tomatoes start to break down.
3. Pour in the low-sodium vegetable broth and bring to a boil. Reduce heat to low and simmer for 15-20 minutes.
4. Remove the saucepan from heat and let it cool slightly.
5. Using a blender or immersion blender, puree the cooked tomatoes, onion, garlic, and broth until smooth.
6. Return the pureed mixture to the saucepan and stir in the Greek yogurt until well combined.
7. Season the soup with salt and pepper to taste.
8. Reheat the soup over low heat until warmed through, stirring occasionally.
9. Serve the creamy tomato and basil soup hot, garnished with fresh basil leaves if desired.

> **Nutritional Info:**
> **Calories: 100 | Protein: 4g | Carbohydrates: 15g | Fat: 4g | Fiber: 3g**

GASTRIC BYPASS COOKBOOK FOR ALL STAGES

Recipe Name:_____

Date: / /   *Time:*_____

Rating: ☆ ☆ ☆ ☆ ☆

S/N	Ingredients	Adjustment

Cooking Experience: _____

_____

_____

_____

Notes:_____

_____

_____

_____

_____

_____

_____

_____

Creamy Zucchini and Avocado Soup

Prep Time: 10 minutes | Cooking Time: 20 minutes | Servings: 2

Ingredients:

- 1 cup chopped zucchini
- 1/4 cup chopped onion
- 1 clove garlic, minced
- 1/2 ripe avocado, peeled and diced
- 1 cup low-sodium vegetable broth
- 1/4 cup Greek yogurt
- 1 tablespoon olive oil
- Salt and pepper, to taste
- Fresh cilantro, for garnish (optional)

Method of Preparation:

1. In a medium saucepan, heat olive oil over medium heat. Add chopped onion and garlic, and sauté until softened, about 5 minutes.
2. Add chopped zucchini to the saucepan. Cook for another 5 minutes until zucchini starts to soften.
3. Pour in the low-sodium vegetable broth and bring to a boil. Reduce heat to low and simmer for 10-15 minutes until zucchini is tender.
4. Remove the saucepan from heat and let it cool slightly.
5. Using a blender or immersion blender, puree the cooked zucchini, onion, garlic, avocado, and broth until smooth.
6. Return the pureed mixture to the saucepan and stir in the Greek yogurt until well combined.
7. Season the soup with salt and pepper to taste.
8. Reheat the soup over low heat until warmed through, stirring occasionally.
9. Serve the creamy zucchini and avocado soup hot, garnished with fresh cilantro if desired.

> **Nutritional Info:**
> Calories: 130 | Protein: 5g | Carbohydrates: 15g | Fat: 7g | Fiber: 5g

GASTRIC BYPASS COOKBOOK FOR ALL STAGES

Recipe Name:_____

Date: / /   *Time:*_____

Rating: ☆ ☆ ☆ ☆ ☆

S/N	Ingredients	Adjustment

Cooking Experience: _____

_____

_____

_____

Notes:_____

_____

_____

_____

_____

_____

_____

CHAPTER THREE
Soft Foods Stage Recipes
Breakfast Recipes

Scrambled Eggs with Avocado

Prep Time: 5 minutes | Cooking Time: 5 minutes | Servings: 2

Ingredients:
- 4 large eggs
- 1 ripe avocado, diced
- 1 tablespoon olive oil
- Salt and pepper, to taste

Method of Preparation:
1. Crack the eggs into a bowl and whisk until well beaten. Season with salt and pepper.
2. Heat olive oil in a non-stick skillet over medium heat.
3. Pour the beaten eggs into the skillet and cook, stirring gently, until scrambled and cooked through, about 3-4 minutes.
4. Remove the skillet from heat and transfer the scrambled eggs to serving plates.
5. Top the scrambled eggs with diced avocado.
6. Serve hot and enjoy!

Nutritional Info:
Calories: 250 | Protein: 14g | Carbohydrates: 9g | Fat: 20g |
Fiber: 7g

GASTRIC BYPASS COOKBOOK FOR ALL STAGES

Recipe Name:_____

Date: / /   *Time:____*

Rating: ☆ ☆ ☆ ☆ ☆

S/N	Ingredients	Adjustment

Cooking Experience: _____

_____

_____

_____

Notes:_____

_____

_____

_____

_____

_____

_____

Greek Yogurt Parfait

Prep Time: 5 minutes | Cooking Time: 0 minutes | Servings: 2

Ingredients:

- 1 cup Greek yogurt
- 1/2 cup fresh berries (such as strawberries, blueberries, or raspberries)
- 2 tablespoons chopped nuts (such as almonds or walnuts)
- 1 tablespoon honey (optional)

Method of Preparation:

1. In two serving glasses or bowls, layer Greek yogurt, fresh berries, and chopped nuts.
2. Drizzle honey over the top if desired.
3. Serve immediately and enjoy!

Nutritional Info:
Calories: 200 | Protein: 15g | Carbohydrates: 20g | Fat: 8g | Fiber: 5g

GASTRIC BYPASS COOKBOOK FOR ALL STAGES

Recipe Name:_____

Date: / /   *Time:*_____

Rating: ☆ ☆ ☆ ☆ ☆

S/N	Ingredients	Adjustment

Cooking Experience: _____

_____

_____

_____

Notes:_____

_____

_____

_____

_____

_____

_____

_____

Cottage Cheese Pancakes

Prep Time: 10 minutes | Cooking Time: 10 minutes | Servings: 2

Ingredients:

- 1 cup cottage cheese
- 2 large eggs
- 1/4 cup almond flour
- 1 teaspoon vanilla extract
- 1 tablespoon olive oil or butter for cooking
- Fresh berries for serving (optional)

Method of Preparation:

1. In a bowl, whisk together cottage cheese, eggs, almond flour, and vanilla extract until smooth.
2. Heat olive oil or butter in a non-stick skillet over medium heat.
3. Spoon the pancake batter onto the skillet to form small pancakes.
4. Cook until bubbles form on the surface, then flip and cook until golden brown on both sides, about 2-3 minutes per side.
5. Repeat with the remaining batter.
6. Serve the pancakes with fresh berries if desired.
7. Enjoy your delicious cottage cheese pancakes!

Nutritional Info:
Calories: 280 | Protein: 20g | Carbohydrates: 10g | Fat: 18g | Fiber: 2g

GASTRIC BYPASS COOKBOOK FOR ALL STAGES

Recipe Name:_____

Date: / /   *Time:_____*

Rating: ☆ ☆ ☆ ☆ ☆

S/N	Ingredients	Adjustment

Cooking Experience: _____
_____
_____
_____

Notes:_____
_____
_____
_____
_____
_____
_____

Soft Scrambled Tofu

Prep Time: 5 minutes | Cooking Time: 10 minutes | Servings: 2

Ingredients:

- 1 block (14 oz) firm tofu, drained and crumbled
- 1 tablespoon olive oil
- 1/4 cup diced bell peppers
- 1/4 cup diced onions
- 1/4 cup chopped spinach
- Salt and pepper, to taste
- Fresh herbs for garnish (optional)

Method of Preparation:

1. Heat olive oil in a non-stick skillet over medium heat.
2. Add diced bell peppers and onions to the skillet and sauté until softened, about 3-4 minutes.
3. Add chopped spinach to the skillet and cook until wilted, about 1-2 minutes.
4. Add crumbled tofu to the skillet and cook, stirring occasionally, until heated through, about 5 minutes.
5. Season with salt and pepper to taste.
6. Garnish with fresh herbs if desired.
7. Serve the soft scrambled tofu hot and enjoy!

Nutritional Info:
Calories: 220 | Protein: 20g | Carbohydrates: 8g | Fat: 12g | Fiber: 2g

GASTRIC BYPASS COOKBOOK FOR ALL STAGES

Recipe Name:_____

Date: / /   *Time:*_____

Rating: ☆ ☆ ☆ ☆ ☆

S/N	Ingredients	Adjustment

Cooking Experience: _____
_____
_____
_____

Notes:_____
_____
_____
_____
_____
_____
_____
_____

Banana Oatmeal Pancakes

Prep Time: 10 minutes | Cooking Time: 10 minutes | Servings: 2

Ingredients:

- 1 ripe banana, mashed
- 2 large eggs
- 1/2 cup rolled oats
- 1/4 teaspoon ground cinnamon
- 1/4 teaspoon vanilla extract
- 1 tablespoon olive oil or butter for cooking
- Maple syrup and sliced bananas for serving (optional)

Method of Preparation:

1. In a bowl, mash the ripe banana until smooth.
2. Add eggs, rolled oats, ground cinnamon, and vanilla extract to the bowl. Mix until well combined.
3. Heat olive oil or butter in a non-stick skillet over medium heat.
4. Pour the pancake batter onto the skillet to form small pancakes.
5. Cook until bubbles form on the surface, then flip and cook until golden brown on both sides, about 2-3 minutes per side.
6. Repeat with the remaining batter.
7. Serve the pancakes with maple syrup and sliced bananas if desired.
8. Enjoy your delicious banana oatmeal pancakes!

Nutritional Info:
Calories: 280 | Protein: 9g | Carbohydrates: 30g | Fat: 14g | Fiber: 4g

GASTRIC BYPASS COOKBOOK FOR ALL STAGES

Recipe Name:_____

Date: / /   *Time:*_____

Rating: ☆ ☆ ☆ ☆ ☆

S/N	Ingredients	Adjustment

Cooking Experience: _____
_____
_____
_____

Notes:_____
_____
_____
_____
_____
_____
_____

Soft Scrambled Eggs with Cheese

Prep Time: 5 minutes | Cooking Time: 5 minutes | Servings: 2

Ingredients:

- 4 large eggs
- 1/4 cup shredded cheddar cheese
- 1 tablespoon olive oil or butter
- Salt and pepper, to taste
- Fresh chives for garnish (optional)

Method of Preparation:

1. Crack the eggs into a bowl and whisk until well beaten. Season with salt and pepper.
2. Heat olive oil or butter in a non-stick skillet over medium heat.
3. Pour the beaten eggs into the skillet and let them cook undisturbed for a few seconds.
4. Using a spatula, gently stir the eggs until they start to set.
5. Sprinkle shredded cheddar cheese over the eggs and continue to stir until the eggs are cooked to your desired consistency.
6. Remove the skillet from heat and transfer the scrambled eggs to serving plates.
7. Garnish with fresh chives if desired.
8. Serve hot and enjoy your soft scrambled eggs with cheese!

Nutritional Info:
Calories: 260 | Protein: 16g | Carbohydrates: 2g | Fat: 20g | Fiber: 0g

GASTRIC BYPASS COOKBOOK FOR ALL STAGES

Recipe Name:_____

Date: / /   *Time:*_____

Rating: ☆ ☆ ☆ ☆ ☆

S/N	Ingredients	Adjustment

Cooking Experience: _____
_____
_____
_____

Notes:_____
_____
_____
_____
_____
_____
_____

Apple Cinnamon Oatmeal

Prep Time: 5 minutes | Cooking Time: 10 minutes | Servings: 2

Ingredients:

- 1 cup old-fashioned rolled oats
- 2 cups water or milk of your choice
- 1 apple, peeled, cored, and diced
- 1/2 teaspoon ground cinnamon
- 1 tablespoon honey or maple syrup (optional)
- Chopped nuts or raisins for topping (optional)

Method of Preparation:

1. In a saucepan, bring water or milk to a boil over medium heat.
2. Stir in rolled oats, diced apple, and ground cinnamon.
3. Reduce heat to low and simmer, stirring occasionally, for about 5-7 minutes until oats are cooked and the mixture thickens.
4. Remove from heat and let it cool slightly.
5. If desired, stir in honey or maple syrup for sweetness.
6. Divide the oatmeal into serving bowls and top with chopped nuts or raisins if desired.
7. Serve warm and enjoy your comforting apple cinnamon oatmeal!

Nutritional Info:
Calories: 250 | Protein: 7g | Carbohydrates: 47g | Fat: 4g | Fiber: 6g

GASTRIC BYPASS COOKBOOK FOR ALL STAGES

Recipe Name:_____

Date: / /   *Time:*_____

Rating: ☆ ☆ ☆ ☆ ☆

S/N	Ingredients	Adjustment

Cooking Experience: _____
_____
_____
_____

Notes:_____
_____
_____
_____
_____
_____
_____

Soft Boiled Eggs with Toast Soldiers

Prep Time: 5 minutes | Cooking Time: 6 minutes | Servings: 2

Ingredients:

- 4 large eggs
- 2 slices whole grain bread
- Salt and pepper, to taste
- Fresh herbs for garnish (optional)

Method of Preparation:

1. Bring a small saucepan of water to a boil over medium-high heat.
2. Gently lower the eggs into the boiling water using a spoon.
3. Reduce heat to low and simmer for exactly 6 minutes for soft boiled eggs.
4. While the eggs are cooking, toast the bread slices until golden brown.
5. Once the eggs are done, immediately transfer them to a bowl of cold water to stop the cooking process.
6. Carefully crack and peel the eggs, then slice off the tops.
7. Season the soft-boiled eggs with salt and pepper.
8. Cut the toasted bread into thin strips to serve as "soldiers" for dipping.
9. Serve the soft-boiled eggs with toast soldiers on the side.
10. Garnish with fresh herbs if desired.
11. Enjoy your delightful soft-boiled eggs with toast soldiers!

Nutritional Info:
Calories: 220 | Protein: 13g | Carbohydrates: 18g | Fat: 10g | Fiber: 4g

GASTRIC BYPASS COOKBOOK FOR ALL STAGES

Recipe Name:_____

Date: / /   *Time:*_____

Rating: ☆ ☆ ☆ ☆ ☆

S/N	Ingredients	Adjustment

Cooking Experience: _____
_____
_____
_____

Notes:_____
_____
_____
_____
_____
_____
_____

Creamy Peanut Butter Banana Smoothie

Prep Time: 5 minutes | Servings: 2

Ingredients:

- 2 ripe bananas, peeled and sliced
- 2 tablespoons natural peanut butter
- 1 cup unsweetened almond milk (or milk of choice)
- 1/2 cup Greek yogurt
- 1 tablespoon honey (optional)
- Ice cubes (optional)

Method of Preparation:

1. In a blender, combine sliced bananas, peanut butter, almond milk, Greek yogurt, and honey.
2. Blend until smooth and creamy. If desired, add ice cubes for a colder smoothie.
3. Pour into glasses and serve immediately.

Nutritional Info:
Calories: 270 | Protein: 10g | Carbohydrates: 30g | Fat: 14g | Fiber: 4g

GASTRIC BYPASS COOKBOOK FOR ALL STAGES

Recipe Name:_____

Date: / /   *Time:*_____

Rating: ☆ ☆ ☆ ☆ ☆

S/N	Ingredients	Adjustment

Cooking Experience: _____
_____
_____
_____

Notes:_____
_____
_____
_____
_____
_____
_____

Soft Scrambled Tofu Breakfast Bowl

Prep Time: 10 minutes | Cooking Time: 10 minutes | Servings: 2

Ingredients:

- 1 block (14 oz) firm tofu, drained and crumbled
- 1 tablespoon olive oil
- 1/4 cup diced bell peppers
- 1/4 cup diced onions
- 1/4 cup chopped spinach
- Salt and pepper, to taste
- 1 avocado, sliced
- Fresh cilantro or parsley for garnish (optional)

Method of Preparation:

1. Heat olive oil in a skillet over medium heat. Add diced bell peppers and onions, and sauté until softened.
2. Add chopped spinach and cook until wilted.
3. Add crumbled tofu to the skillet and cook, stirring occasionally, until heated through.
4. Season with salt and pepper to taste.
5. Divide the scrambled tofu mixture into serving bowls.
6. Top with sliced avocado and garnish with fresh cilantro or parsley if desired.
7. Serve hot and enjoy your soft scrambled tofu breakfast bowl!

> *Nutritional Info:*
> *Calories: 280 | Protein: 15g | Carbohydrates: 12g | Fat: 20g | Fiber: 7g*

GASTRIC BYPASS COOKBOOK FOR ALL STAGES

Recipe Name:_____

Date: / /   *Time:*_____

Rating: ☆ ☆ ☆ ☆ ☆

S/N	Ingredients	Adjustment

Cooking Experience: _____
_____
_____
_____

Notes:_____
_____
_____
_____
_____
_____
_____

Lunch Recipes

Turkey and Avocado Wrap

Prep Time: 10 minutes | Cooking Time: 0 minutes | Servings: 2

Ingredients:

- 4 slices deli turkey breast
- 1 ripe avocado, sliced
- 2 large lettuce leaves
- 2 whole grain tortillas or wraps
- Mustard or mayo, for spreading (optional)
- Salt and pepper, to taste

Method of Preparation:

1. Lay out the tortillas or wraps on a clean surface.
2. Spread mustard or mayo (if using) on the tortillas.
3. Place 2 slices of turkey breast on each tortilla.
4. Top with avocado slices and lettuce leaves.
5. Season with salt and pepper to taste.
6. Roll up the tortillas tightly into wraps.
7. Slice in half if desired and serve immediately.

Nutritional Info:
Calories: 320 | Protein: 20g | Carbohydrates: 25g | Fat: 16g | Fiber: 8g

GASTRIC BYPASS COOKBOOK FOR ALL STAGES

Recipe Name:_____

Date: / /   *Time:*_____

Rating: ☆ ☆ ☆ ☆ ☆

S/N	Ingredients	Adjustment

Cooking Experience: _____
_____
_____
_____

Notes:_____
_____
_____
_____
_____
_____
_____

Salmon Salad

Prep Time: 10 minutes | Cooking Time: 10 minutes | Servings: 2

Ingredients:
- 2 salmon fillets (about 4 oz each)
- 4 cups mixed greens
- 1/2 cup cherry tomatoes, halved
- 1/4 cup cucumber, sliced
- 2 tablespoons balsamic vinaigrette
- Salt and pepper, to taste

Method of Preparation:
1. Season salmon fillets with salt and pepper.
2. Heat a non-stick skillet over medium heat. Add salmon fillets and cook for about 4-5 minutes on each side until cooked through.
3. In a large mixing bowl, toss mixed greens, cherry tomatoes, and cucumber with balsamic vinaigrette.
4. Divide the salad mixture onto serving plates.
5. Top each salad with a cooked salmon fillet.
6. Serve immediately.

Nutritional Info:
Calories: 290 | Protein: 25g | Carbohydrates: 10g | Fat: 16g | Fiber: 4g

GASTRIC BYPASS COOKBOOK FOR ALL STAGES

Recipe Name:_____

Date: / /   *Time:*_____

Rating: ☆ ☆ ☆ ☆ ☆

S/N	Ingredients	Adjustment

Cooking Experience: _____
_____
_____
_____

Notes:_____
_____
_____
_____
_____
_____
_____

Chicken and Avocado Salad

Prep Time: 10 minutes | Cooking Time: 10 minutes | Servings: 2

Ingredients:

- 2 boneless, skinless chicken breasts
- Salt and pepper, to taste
- 4 cups mixed greens
- 1 avocado, diced
- 1/4 cup cherry tomatoes, halved
- 1/4 cup cucumber, sliced
- 2 tablespoons olive oil
- 1 tablespoon balsamic vinegar
- 1 teaspoon Dijon mustard (optional)

Method of Preparation:

1. Season chicken breasts with salt and pepper.
2. Heat a non-stick skillet over medium heat. Add chicken breasts and cook for about 4-5 minutes on each side until cooked through.
3. In a large mixing bowl, toss mixed greens, diced avocado, cherry tomatoes, and cucumber.
4. In a small bowl, whisk together olive oil, balsamic vinegar, and Dijon mustard (if using) to make the dressing.
5. Divide the salad mixture onto serving plates.
6. Slice the cooked chicken breasts and place on top of each salad.
7. Drizzle the dressing over the salads.
8. Serve immediately.

Nutritional Info:
Calories: 320 | Protein: 30g | Carbohydrates: 12g | Fat: 18g |
Fiber: 7g

GASTRIC BYPASS COOKBOOK FOR ALL STAGES

Recipe Name:_____

Date: / /   *Time:*_____

Rating: ☆ ☆ ☆ ☆ ☆

S/N	Ingredients	Adjustment

Cooking Experience: _____
_____
_____
_____

Notes:_____
_____
_____
_____
_____
_____
_____

Tuna Salad Lettuce Wraps

Prep Time: 10 minutes | Cooking Time: 0 minutes | Servings: 2

Ingredients:

- 2 cans (5 oz each) tuna, drained
- 1/4 cup diced celery
- 1/4 cup diced red onion
- 2 tablespoons Greek yogurt
- 1 tablespoon lemon juice
- Salt and pepper, to taste
- 4 large lettuce leaves

Method of Preparation:

1. In a mixing bowl, combine drained tuna, diced celery, diced red onion, Greek yogurt, and lemon juice.
2. Season with salt and pepper to taste and mix well.
3. Place a spoonful of the tuna salad onto each lettuce leaf.
4. Roll up the lettuce leaves to form wraps.
5. Serve immediately.

Nutritional Info:
Calories: 200 | Protein: 30g | Carbohydrates: 6g | Fat: 6g | Fiber: 2g

GASTRIC BYPASS COOKBOOK FOR ALL STAGES

Recipe Name:

Date: / /   *Time:*_____

Rating: ☆ ☆ ☆ ☆ ☆

S/N	Ingredients	Adjustment

Cooking Experience: _____

_____

_____

_____

Notes:_____

_____

_____

_____

_____

_____

_____

Egg Salad Lettuce Wraps

Prep Time: 10 minutes | Cooking Time: 10 minutes | Servings: 2

Ingredients:

- 4 hard-boiled eggs, chopped
- 1/4 cup diced celery
- 1/4 cup diced red onion
- 2 tablespoons Greek yogurt
- 1 tablespoon Dijon mustard
- Salt and pepper, to taste
- 4 large lettuce leaves

Method of Preparation:

1. In a mixing bowl, combine chopped hard-boiled eggs, diced celery, diced red onion, Greek yogurt, and Dijon mustard.
2. Season with salt and pepper to taste and mix well.
3. Place a spoonful of the egg salad onto each lettuce leaf.
4. Roll up the lettuce leaves to form wraps.
5. Serve immediately.

Nutritional Info:
Calories: 220 | Protein: 16g | Carbohydrates: 6g | Fat: 14g | Fiber: 2g

Recipe Name:_____

Date: / /   *Time:*____

Rating: ☆ ☆ ☆ ☆ ☆

S/N	Ingredients	Adjustment

Cooking Experience: _____

_____

_____

_____

Notes:_____

_____

_____

_____

_____

_____

_____

Quinoa and Vegetable Salad

Prep Time: 15 minutes | Cooking Time: 15 minutes | Servings: 2

Ingredients:

- 1/2 cup quinoa
- 1 cup water or low-sodium vegetable broth
- 1/2 cup diced cucumber
- 1/2 cup diced bell peppers
- 1/4 cup chopped parsley
- 2 tablespoons olive oil
- 1 tablespoon lemon juice
- Salt and pepper, to taste

Method of Preparation:

1. Rinse quinoa under cold water.
2. In a saucepan, combine quinoa and water or vegetable broth.
3. Bring to a boil, then reduce heat, cover, and simmer for 12-15 minutes until quinoa is cooked and liquid is absorbed. Remove from heat and let it cool.
4. In a large mixing bowl, combine cooked quinoa, diced cucumber, diced bell peppers, and chopped parsley.
5. In a small bowl, whisk together olive oil and lemon juice to make the dressing.
6. Pour the dressing over the quinoa and vegetable mixture. Toss until well combined.
7. Season with salt and pepper to taste.
8. Serve immediately or chill in the refrigerator for later use.

Nutritional Info:
Calories: 280 | Protein: 8g | Carbohydrates: 30g | Fat: 14g | Fiber: 5g

GASTRIC BYPASS COOKBOOK FOR ALL STAGES

Recipe Name:_____

Date: / /   *Time:*_____

Rating: ☆ ☆ ☆ ☆ ☆

S/N	Ingredients	Adjustment

Cooking Experience: _____
_____
_____
_____

Notes:_____
_____
_____
_____
_____
_____
_____

Avocado Tuna Salad

Prep Time: 10 minutes | Cooking Time: 0 minutes | Servings: 2

Ingredients:

- 2 cans (5 oz each) tuna, drained
- 1 ripe avocado, mashed
- 1/4 cup diced celery
- 1/4 cup diced red onion
- 1 tablespoon lemon juice
- Salt and pepper, to taste
- Lettuce leaves or whole grain bread for serving

Method of Preparation:

1. In a mixing bowl, combine drained tuna, mashed avocado, diced celery, diced red onion, and lemon juice.
2. Season with salt and pepper to taste and mix well.
3. Serve the avocado tuna salad on lettuce leaves as wraps or spread on whole grain bread to make sandwiches.
4. Enjoy your delicious and creamy avocado tuna salad!

Nutritional Info:
Calories: 280 | Protein: 30g | Carbohydrates: 10g | Fat: 14g | Fiber: 6g

GASTRIC BYPASS COOKBOOK FOR ALL STAGES

Recipe Name:_____

Date: / /   *Time:*_____

Rating: ☆ ☆ ☆ ☆ ☆

S/N	Ingredients	Adjustment

Cooking Experience: _____
_____
_____
_____

Notes:_____
_____
_____
_____
_____
_____
_____

Turkey and Hummus Wrap

Prep Time: 10 minutes | Cooking Time: 0 minutes | Servings: 2

Ingredients:

- 4 slices deli turkey breast
- 4 tablespoons hummus
- 1/2 cup shredded lettuce
- 1/4 cup shredded carrots
- 2 whole grain tortillas or wraps

Method of Preparation:

1. Lay out the tortillas or wraps on a clean surface.
2. Spread 2 tablespoons of hummus evenly on each tortilla.
3. Place 2 slices of turkey breast on each tortilla.
4. Top with shredded lettuce and shredded carrots.
5. Roll up the tortillas tightly into wraps.
6. Slice in half if desired and serve immediately.
7. Enjoy your flavorful and satisfying turkey and hummus wraps!

Nutritional Info:
Calories: 250 | Protein: 20g | Carbohydrates: 25g | Fat: 10g |
Fiber: 6g

GASTRIC BYPASS COOKBOOK FOR ALL STAGES

Recipe Name:_____

Date: / /   *Time:*_____

Rating: ☆ ☆ ☆ ☆ ☆

S/N	Ingredients	Adjustment

Cooking Experience: _____
_____
_____
_____

Notes:_____
_____
_____
_____
_____
_____
_____

Chicken and Quinoa Bowl

Prep Time: 10 minutes | Cooking Time: 15 minutes | Servings: 2

Ingredients:

- 2 boneless, skinless chicken breasts
- Salt and pepper, to taste
- 1/2 cup cooked quinoa
- 1/2 cup steamed mixed vegetables (such as carrots, broccoli, and cauliflower)
- 2 tablespoons Greek yogurt
- 1 tablespoon lemon juice
- Fresh parsley or cilantro for garnish (optional)

Method of Preparation:

1. Season chicken breasts with salt and pepper.
2. Heat a non-stick skillet over medium heat. Add chicken breasts and cook for about 4-5 minutes on each side until cooked through.
3. In a mixing bowl, combine cooked quinoa and steamed mixed vegetables.
4. In a small bowl, whisk together Greek yogurt and lemon juice to make the dressing.
5. Divide the quinoa and vegetable mixture onto serving bowls.
6. Slice the cooked chicken breasts and place on top of each bowl.
7. Drizzle the dressing over the bowls.
8. Garnish with fresh parsley or cilantro if desired.
9. Serve immediately.

Nutritional Info:
Calories: 300 | Protein: 30g | Carbohydrates: 20g | Fat: 10g |
Fiber: 4g

GASTRIC BYPASS COOKBOOK FOR ALL STAGES

Recipe Name:_____

Date: / /   *Time:*_____

Rating: ☆ ☆ ☆ ☆ ☆

S/N	Ingredients	Adjustment

Cooking Experience: _____
_____
_____
_____

Notes:_____
_____
_____
_____
_____
_____
_____

Shrimp and Avocado Salad

Prep Time: 10 minutes | Cooking Time: 5 minutes | Servings: 2

Ingredients:

- 1/2 lb. shrimp, peeled and deveined
- Salt and pepper, to taste
- 4 cups mixed greens
- 1 avocado, diced
- 1/4 cup cherry tomatoes, halved
- 2 tablespoons olive oil
- 1 tablespoon balsamic vinegar
- Fresh lemon wedges for serving (optional)

Method of Preparation:

1. Season shrimp with salt and pepper.
2. Heat olive oil in a skillet over medium heat. Add shrimp and cook for about 2-3 minutes on each side until pink and cooked through.
3. In a large mixing bowl, toss mixed greens, diced avocado, and cherry tomatoes.
4. In a small bowl, whisk together olive oil and balsamic vinegar to make the dressing.
5. Divide the salad mixture onto serving plates.
6. Arrange cooked shrimp on top of each salad.
7. Drizzle the dressing over the salads.
8. Serve immediately with fresh lemon wedges if desired.

Nutritional Info:
Calories: 280 | Protein: 25g | Carbohydrates: 12g | Fat: 16g | Fiber: 7g

GASTRIC BYPASS COOKBOOK FOR ALL STAGES

Recipe Name:_____

Date: / /   *Time:*_____

Rating: ☆ ☆ ☆ ☆ ☆

S/N	Ingredients	Adjustment

Cooking Experience: _____

_____

_____

_____

Notes:_____

_____

_____

_____

_____

_____

_____

Dinner Recipes

Baked Salmon with Mashed Sweet Potatoes

Prep Time: 10 minutes | Cooking Time: 20 minutes | Servings: 2

Ingredients:

- 2 salmon fillets (about 4 oz each)
- Salt and pepper, to taste
- 2 medium sweet potatoes, peeled and diced
- 1 tablespoon olive oil
- 2 tablespoons unsweetened almond milk
- 1 tablespoon chopped fresh parsley (optional)

Method of Preparation:

1. Preheat the oven to 400°F (200°C).
2. Season salmon fillets with salt and pepper on both sides.
3. Place salmon fillets on a baking sheet lined with parchment paper.
4. Bake in the preheated oven for about 15-20 minutes until salmon is cooked through and flakes easily with a fork.
5. While the salmon is baking, boil diced sweet potatoes in a pot of water until tender, about 10-15 minutes.
6. Drain the sweet potatoes and transfer them to a mixing bowl.
7. Mash the sweet potatoes using a potato masher or fork.
8. Stir in olive oil and almond milk until smooth and creamy.
9. Season with salt and pepper to taste.
10. Serve the baked salmon with mashed sweet potatoes.
11. Garnish with chopped fresh parsley if desired.
12. Enjoy your delicious and nutritious dinner!

Nutritional Info: Calories: 350 | Protein: 25g | Carbohydrates: 30g | Fat: 15g | Fiber: 5g

GASTRIC BYPASS COOKBOOK FOR ALL STAGES

Recipe Name:_____

Date: / / *Time:*_____

Rating: ☆ ☆ ☆ ☆ ☆

S/N	Ingredients	Adjustment

Cooking Experience: _____
_____
_____
_____

Notes:_____
_____
_____
_____
_____
_____
_____
_____

Turkey Meatballs with Zucchini Noodles

Prep Time: 15 minutes | Cooking Time: 20 minutes | Servings: 2

Ingredients:

- 1/2 lb. ground turkey
- 1/4 cup almond flour
- 1/4 cup grated Parmesan cheese
- 1 egg
- 2 cloves garlic, minced
- 1 tablespoon chopped fresh parsley
- Salt and pepper, to taste
- 2 medium zucchini, spiralized into noodles
- 1 tablespoon olive oil
- Marinara sauce, for serving (optional)

Method of Preparation:

1. Preheat the oven to 400°F (200°C).
2. In a mixing bowl, combine ground turkey, almond flour, Parmesan cheese, egg, minced garlic, chopped parsley, salt, and pepper. Mix until well combined.
3. Shape the turkey mixture into meatballs and place them on a baking sheet lined with parchment paper.
4. Bake in the preheated oven for about 15-20 minutes until meatballs are cooked through.
5. While the meatballs are baking, heat olive oil in a skillet over medium heat.
6. Add spiralized zucchini noodles to the skillet and sauté for 3-4 minutes until tender.
7. Season the zucchini noodles with salt and pepper to taste.
8. Serve the turkey meatballs with zucchini noodles.
9. Top with marinara sauce if desired.
10. Enjoy your flavorful and satisfying dinner!

> **Nutritional Info:**
> Calories: 320 | Protein: 25g | Carbohydrates: 10g | Fat: 20g |
> Fiber: 3g

GASTRIC BYPASS COOKBOOK FOR ALL STAGES

Recipe Name:

Date: / /   *Time:*_____

Rating: ☆ ☆ ☆ ☆ ☆

S/N	Ingredients	Adjustment

Cooking Experience: _____

_____

_____

_____

Notes:_____

_____

_____

_____

_____

_____

_____

Baked Chicken Breast with Roasted Vegetables

Prep Time: 15 minutes | Cooking Time: 25 minutes | Servings: 2

Ingredients:

- 2 boneless, skinless chicken breasts
- Salt and pepper, to taste
- 1 tablespoon olive oil
- 1 medium zucchini, sliced
- 1 medium yellow squash, sliced
- 1 red bell pepper, sliced
- 1 yellow bell pepper, sliced
- 1 small red onion, sliced
- 2 cloves garlic, minced
- 1 teaspoon dried Italian seasoning
- Fresh parsley for garnish (optional)

Method of Preparation:

1. Preheat the oven to 400°F (200°C).
2. Season chicken breasts with salt and pepper on both sides.
3. Heat olive oil in an oven-safe skillet over medium-high heat. Add chicken breasts and sear for 2-3 minutes on each side until golden brown.
4. In a mixing bowl, combine sliced zucchini, yellow squash, red bell pepper, yellow bell pepper, red onion, minced garlic, dried Italian seasoning, salt, and pepper. Toss to coat.
5. Transfer the skillet with seared chicken breasts to the oven. Arrange the seasoned vegetables around the chicken.
6. Bake in the preheated oven for about 20-25 minutes until chicken is cooked through and vegetables are tender.
7. Remove from the oven and let it rest for a few minutes.
8. Serve the baked chicken breast with roasted vegetables.
9. Garnish with fresh parsley if desired.

10. Enjoy your flavorful and healthy dinner!

> **Nutritional Info:**
> **Calories: 320 | Protein: 30g | Carbohydrates: 15g | Fat: 15g | Fiber: 5g**

GASTRIC BYPASS COOKBOOK FOR ALL STAGES

Recipe Name:_____

Date: / /   *Time:*_____

Rating: ☆ ☆ ☆ ☆ ☆

S/N	Ingredients	Adjustment

Cooking Experience: _____

_____
_____
_____

Notes:_____

_____
_____
_____
_____
_____
_____
_____

Lentil Soup

Prep Time: 10 minutes | Cooking Time: 30 minutes | Servings: 4

Ingredients:

- 1 cup dried lentils, rinsed and drained
- 4 cups low-sodium chicken or vegetable broth
- 1 onion, chopped
- 2 carrots, chopped
- 2 celery stalks, chopped
- 2 cloves garlic, minced
- 1 teaspoon dried thyme
- 1 bay leaf
- Salt and pepper, to taste
- Fresh parsley for garnish (optional)

Method of Preparation:

1. In a large pot, combine dried lentils, chicken or vegetable broth, chopped onion, carrots, celery, minced garlic, dried thyme, bay leaf, salt, and pepper.
2. Bring the mixture to a boil over medium-high heat. Reduce heat to low, cover, and simmer for about 25-30 minutes until lentils and vegetables are tender.
3. Remove the bay leaf from the soup and discard.
4. Using an immersion blender or regular blender, blend half of the soup until smooth. Alternatively, you can leave the soup chunky if desired.
5. Serve the lentil soup hot.
6. Garnish with fresh parsley if desired.
7. Enjoy your comforting and nutritious dinner!

Nutritional Info:
Calories: 250 | Protein: 15g | Carbohydrates: 40g | Fat: 2g | Fiber: 15g

GASTRIC BYPASS COOKBOOK FOR ALL STAGES

Recipe Name:_____

Date: / /   *Time:*_____

Rating: ☆ ☆ ☆ ☆ ☆

S/N	Ingredients	Adjustment

Cooking Experience: _____
_____
_____
_____

Notes:_____
_____
_____
_____
_____
_____
_____

Baked Cod with Roasted Vegetables

Prep Time: 15 minutes | Cooking Time: 20 minutes | Servings: 2

Ingredients:

- 2 cod fillets (about 4 oz each)
- Salt and pepper, to taste
- 1 tablespoon olive oil
- 1 cup cherry tomatoes
- 1 cup sliced mushrooms
- 1 cup chopped broccoli florets
- 2 cloves garlic, minced
- 1 teaspoon dried thyme
- Lemon wedges for serving (optional)
- Fresh parsley for garnish (optional)

Method of Preparation:

1. Preheat the oven to 400°F (200°C).
2. Season cod fillets with salt and pepper on both sides.
3. Place cod fillets on a baking sheet lined with parchment paper.
4. In a mixing bowl, combine cherry tomatoes, sliced mushrooms, chopped broccoli florets, minced garlic, dried thyme, olive oil, salt, and pepper. Toss to coat.
5. Arrange the seasoned vegetables around the cod fillets on the baking sheet.
6. Bake in the preheated oven for about 15-20 minutes until cod is cooked through and flakes easily with a fork.
7. Remove from the oven and let it rest for a few minutes.
8. Serve the baked cod with roasted vegetables.
9. Garnish with fresh parsley and lemon wedges if desired.
10. Enjoy your flavorful and nutritious dinner!

Nutritional Info:
Calories: 280 | Protein: 25g | Carbohydrates: 10g | Fat: 15g |
Fiber: 4g

GASTRIC BYPASS COOKBOOK FOR ALL STAGES

Recipe Name:_____

Date: / /   *Time:*_____

Rating: ☆ ☆ ☆ ☆ ☆

S/N	Ingredients	Adjustment

Cooking Experience: _____
_____
_____
_____

Notes:_____
_____
_____
_____
_____
_____
_____
_____

Turkey Chili

Prep Time: 15 minutes | Cooking Time: 30 minutes | Servings: 4

Ingredients:

- 1 lb. ground turkey
- 1 onion, chopped
- 2 cloves garlic, minced
- 1 bell pepper, diced
- 1 can (14 oz) diced tomatoes
- 1 can (15 oz) kidney beans, drained and rinsed
- 1 cup low-sodium chicken broth
- 2 tablespoons tomato paste
- 1 tablespoon chili powder
- 1 teaspoon ground cumin
- Salt and pepper, to taste
- Fresh cilantro for garnish (optional)
- Greek yogurt for serving (optional)

Method of Preparation:

1. In a large pot, heat olive oil over medium heat. Add ground turkey and cook until browned, breaking it up with a spoon.
2. Add chopped onion, minced garlic, and diced bell pepper to the pot. Cook until vegetables are softened.
3. Stir in diced tomatoes, kidney beans, chicken broth, tomato paste, chili powder, ground cumin, salt, and pepper.
4. Bring the chili to a boil, then reduce heat to low. Simmer for about 20-25 minutes, stirring occasionally.
5. Adjust seasoning to taste with salt and pepper.
6. Serve the turkey chili hot.
7. Garnish with fresh cilantro and a dollop of Greek yogurt if desired.
8. Enjoy your hearty and flavorful dinner!

Nutritional Info:
Calories: 300 | Protein: 25g | Carbohydrates: 20g | Fat: 10g | Fiber: 6g

GASTRIC BYPASS COOKBOOK FOR ALL STAGES

Recipe Name:_____

Date: / /   *Time:_____*

Rating: ☆ ☆ ☆ ☆ ☆

S/N	Ingredients	Adjustment

Cooking Experience: _____
_____
_____
_____

Notes:_____
_____
_____
_____
_____
_____
_____

Turkey and Vegetable Stir-Fry

Prep Time: 15 minutes | Cooking Time: 15 minutes | Servings: 2

Ingredients:

- 1/2 lb. ground turkey
- 1 tablespoon olive oil
- 1 small onion, thinly sliced
- 1 bell pepper, thinly sliced
- 1 cup broccoli florets
- 1 cup sliced mushrooms
- 2 cloves garlic, minced
- 2 tablespoons low-sodium soy sauce
- 1 tablespoon hoisin sauce
- 1 teaspoon sesame oil
- Cooked brown rice, for serving (optional)
- Sesame seeds for garnish (optional)
- Green onions for garnish (optional)

Method of Preparation:

1. Heat olive oil in a large skillet or wok over medium-high heat.
2. Add ground turkey and cook until browned, breaking it up with a spoon.
3. Add sliced onion, bell pepper, broccoli florets, and sliced mushrooms to the skillet. Cook for 3-4 minutes until vegetables are tender-crisp.
4. Stir in minced garlic and cook for an additional minute.
5. In a small bowl, whisk together low-sodium soy sauce, hoisin sauce, and sesame oil.
6. Pour the sauce mixture over the turkey and vegetables in the skillet. Stir to combine and coat everything evenly with the sauce.
7. Cook for another 2-3 minutes until heated through.

8. Serve the turkey and vegetable stir-fry hot, with cooked brown rice if desired.
9. Garnish with sesame seeds and chopped green onions if desired.
10. Enjoy your flavorful and nutritious dinner!

Nutritional Info:
Calories: 280 | Protein: 20g | Carbohydrates: 15g | Fat: 15g |
Fiber: 4g

GASTRIC BYPASS COOKBOOK FOR ALL STAGES

Recipe Name:_____

Date: /   /   *Time:*_____

Rating: ☆ ☆ ☆ ☆ ☆

S/N	Ingredients	Adjustment

Cooking Experience: _____
_____
_____
_____

Notes:_____
_____
_____
_____
_____
_____
_____

Vegetable Frittata

Prep Time: 10 minutes | Cooking Time: 20 minutes | Servings: 4

Ingredients:

- 6 eggs
- 1/4 cup milk or unsweetened almond milk
- Salt and pepper, to taste
- 1 tablespoon olive oil
- 1 small onion, diced
- 1 bell pepper, diced
- 1 cup sliced mushrooms
- 1 cup baby spinach
- 1/4 cup grated Parmesan cheese
- Fresh parsley for garnish (optional)

Method of Preparation:

1. Preheat the oven to 350°F (175°C).
2. In a mixing bowl, whisk together eggs, milk, salt, and pepper until well combined.
3. Heat olive oil in an oven-safe skillet over medium heat.
4. Add diced onion, diced bell pepper, and sliced mushrooms to the skillet. Cook for 3-4 minutes until vegetables are softened.
5. Stir in baby spinach and cook for another 1-2 minutes until wilted.
6. Pour the egg mixture evenly over the vegetables in the skillet.
7. Sprinkle grated Parmesan cheese on top of the frittata.
8. Transfer the skillet to the preheated oven and bake for about 15-20 minutes until the frittata is set and golden brown on top.
9. Remove from the oven and let it cool slightly.

10. Slice the frittata into wedges, garnish with fresh parsley if desired, and serve.
11. Enjoy your delicious and hearty vegetable frittata!

> ***Nutritional Info:***
> ***Calories: 200 | Protein: 15g | Carbohydrates: 8g | Fat: 12g | Fiber: 2g***

GASTRIC BYPASS COOKBOOK FOR ALL STAGES

Recipe Name:_____

Date: / /   *Time:*_____

Rating: ☆ ☆ ☆ ☆ ☆

S/N	Ingredients	Adjustment

Cooking Experience: _____
_____
_____
_____

Notes:_____
_____
_____
_____
_____
_____
_____
_____

Lemon Herb Baked Tilapia

Prep Time: 10 minutes | Cooking Time: 15 minutes | Servings: 2

Ingredients:

- 2 tilapia fillets (about 4 oz each)
- Salt and pepper, to taste
- 1 tablespoon olive oil
- 1 lemon, thinly sliced
- 2 cloves garlic, minced
- 1 teaspoon dried thyme
- 1 teaspoon dried rosemary
- Fresh parsley for garnish (optional)

Method of Preparation:

1. Preheat the oven to 400°F (200°C).
2. Season tilapia fillets with salt and pepper on both sides.
3. Drizzle olive oil on a baking dish or sheet pan and spread it evenly.
4. Place tilapia fillets on the prepared baking dish.
5. Arrange lemon slices on top of the tilapia fillets.
6. Sprinkle minced garlic, dried thyme, and dried rosemary over the tilapia fillets.
7. Bake in the preheated oven for about 12-15 minutes until tilapia is cooked through and flakes easily with a fork.
8. Remove from the oven and let it rest for a few minutes.
9. Serve the lemon herb baked tilapia hot.
10. Garnish with fresh parsley if desired.
11. Enjoy your flavorful and light dinner!

Nutritional Info:
Calories: 180 | Protein: 25g | Carbohydrates: 3g | Fat: 8g | Fiber: 1g

GASTRIC BYPASS COOKBOOK FOR ALL STAGES

Recipe Name:_____

Date: / /   *Time:*_____

Rating: ☆ ☆ ☆ ☆ ☆

S/N	Ingredients	Adjustment

Cooking Experience: _____
_____
_____
_____

Notes:_____
_____
_____
_____
_____
_____
_____
_____

Eggplant Parmesan

Prep Time: 20 minutes | Cooking Time: 30 minutes | Servings: 2

Ingredients:

- 1 large eggplant, thinly sliced
- Salt and pepper, to taste
- 1 cup marinara sauce
- 1/2 cup shredded mozzarella cheese
- 1/4 cup grated Parmesan cheese
- Fresh basil leaves for garnish (optional)

Method of Preparation:

1. Preheat the oven to 375°F (190°C).
2. Sprinkle salt over the eggplant slices and let them sit for about 10 minutes to release excess moisture. Pat dry with paper towels.
3. Season eggplant slices with salt and pepper.
4. In a baking dish, spread a thin layer of marinara sauce.
5. Arrange a layer of eggplant slices on top of the marinara sauce.
6. Spoon more marinara sauce over the eggplant slices.
7. Sprinkle shredded mozzarella cheese and grated Parmesan cheese over the sauce.
8. Repeat the layers until all eggplant slices are used, ending with cheese on top.
9. Cover the baking dish with aluminum foil and bake in the preheated oven for about 25 minutes.
10. Remove the foil and bake for an additional 5 minutes until the cheese is bubbly and golden brown.
11. Remove from the oven and let it cool slightly.
12. Garnish with fresh basil leaves if desired.
13. Serve the eggplant Parmesan hot.
14. Enjoy your comforting and flavorful dinner!

> **Nutritional Info:**
> **Calories: 250 | Protein: 12g | Carbohydrates: 20g | Fat: 15g | Fiber: 8g**

GASTRIC BYPASS COOKBOOK FOR ALL STAGES

Recipe Name:_____

Date: / /   *Time:*_____

Rating: ☆ ☆ ☆ ☆ ☆

S/N	Ingredients	Adjustment

Cooking Experience: _____
_____
_____
_____

Notes:_____
_____
_____
_____
_____
_____
_____
_____

GASTRIC BYPASS COOKBOOK FOR ALL STAGES

CHAPTER FOUR
Regular Foods Stage Recipes
Breakfast Recipes

Veggie Omelette

Prep Time: 10 minutes | Cooking Time: 10 minutes | Servings: 2

Ingredients:

- 4 large eggs
- 1/4 cup diced bell peppers
- 1/4 cup diced tomatoes
- 1/4 cup diced onions
- 1/4 cup chopped spinach
- Salt and pepper, to taste
- 1 tablespoon olive oil
- 1/4 cup shredded cheese (optional)
- Fresh herbs for garnish (optional)

Method of Preparation:

1. In a mixing bowl, beat the eggs until well combined. Season with salt and pepper.
2. Heat olive oil in a non-stick skillet over medium heat.
3. Add diced bell peppers, tomatoes, onions, and chopped spinach to the skillet. Cook for 2-3 minutes until softened.
4. Pour the beaten eggs over the cooked vegetables in the skillet.
5. Cook for 3-4 minutes until the edges start to set.
6. If using shredded cheese, sprinkle it evenly over one half of the omelette.
7. Using a spatula, fold the omelette in half to cover the cheese.
8. Cook for another 2-3 minutes until the cheese is melted and the omelette is cooked through.

9. Slide the omelette onto a plate and garnish with fresh herbs if desired.
10. Serve hot and enjoy your delicious veggie omelette!

Nutritional Info:
Calories: 250 | Protein: 15g | Carbohydrates: 5g | Fat: 18g | Fiber: 2g

GASTRIC BYPASS COOKBOOK FOR ALL STAGES

Recipe Name:_____

Date: / /   *Time:*_____

Rating: ☆ ☆ ☆ ☆ ☆

S/N	Ingredients	Adjustment

Cooking Experience: _____
_____
_____
_____

Notes:_____
_____
_____
_____
_____
_____
_____
_____

Greek Yogurt Parfait

Prep Time: 5 minutes | Cooking Time: 0 minutes | Servings: 2

Ingredients:

- 1 cup Greek yogurt
- 1/2 cup mixed berries (such as strawberries, blueberries, and raspberries)
- 1/4 cup granola
- 1 tablespoon honey or maple syrup (optional)
- Fresh mint leaves for garnish (optional)

Method of Preparation:

1. In two serving glasses or bowls, layer Greek yogurt, mixed berries, and granola.
2. Repeat the layers until the glasses or bowls are filled.
3. Drizzle honey or maple syrup over the top if desired.
4. Garnish with fresh mint leaves.
5. Serve immediately and enjoy your refreshing Greek yogurt parfait!

Nutritional Info:
Calories: 200 | Protein: 15g | Carbohydrates: 25g | Fat: 8g | Fiber: 3g

GASTRIC BYPASS COOKBOOK FOR ALL STAGES

Recipe Name:_____

Date: / /   *Time:_____*

Rating: ☆ ☆ ☆ ☆ ☆

S/N	Ingredients	Adjustment

Cooking Experience: _____
_____
_____
_____

Notes:_____
_____
_____
_____
_____
_____
_____

Avocado Toast with Poached Egg

Prep Time: 10 minutes | Cooking Time: 5 minutes | Servings: 2

Ingredients:

- 2 slices whole grain bread
- 1 ripe avocado
- Salt and pepper, to taste
- 2 eggs
- 1 tablespoon white vinegar
- Red pepper flakes for garnish (optional)
- Fresh chives for garnish (optional)

Method of Preparation:

1. Toast the slices of whole grain bread until golden brown.
2. While the bread is toasting, halve the avocado and remove the pit. Scoop the avocado flesh into a bowl and mash it with a fork. Season with salt and pepper to taste.
3. In a small pot, bring water to a simmer. Add white vinegar to the water.
4. Crack one egg into a small bowl. Using a spoon, create a gentle whirlpool in the simmering water and carefully slide the egg into the center of the whirlpool. Repeat with the second egg.
5. Poach the eggs for about 3-4 minutes until the whites are set but the yolks are still runny.
6. Remove the poached eggs with a slotted spoon and drain excess water on a paper towel.
7. Spread mashed avocado evenly onto each slice of toasted bread.
8. Top each avocado toast with a poached egg.
9. Garnish with red pepper flakes and fresh chives if desired.
10. Serve immediately and enjoy your delicious avocado toast with poached egg!

Nutritional Info:
Calories: 250 | Protein: 12g | Carbohydrates: 20g | Fat: 15g | Fiber: 6g

GASTRIC BYPASS COOKBOOK FOR ALL STAGES

Recipe Name:_____

Date: / /   *Time:*_____

Rating: ☆ ☆ ☆ ☆ ☆

S/N	Ingredients	Adjustment

Cooking Experience: _____

_____

_____

_____

Notes:_____

_____

_____

_____

_____

_____

_____

_____

Turkey and Cheese Breakfast Wrap

Prep Time: 10 minutes | Cooking Time: 5 minutes | Servings: 2

Ingredients:

- 2 large whole grain tortillas
- 4 slices turkey breast
- 2 slices cheese (such as cheddar or Swiss)
- 1/2 avocado, sliced
- 1/4 cup baby spinach leaves
- 2 tablespoons salsa (optional)
- Salt and pepper, to taste

Method of Preparation:

1. Heat a non-stick skillet over medium heat.
2. Place one tortilla in the skillet and warm it for about 1 minute on each side.
3. Remove the tortilla from the skillet and place it on a flat surface.
4. Layer two slices of turkey breast, one slice of cheese, sliced avocado, and baby spinach leaves on one half of the tortilla.
5. Season with salt and pepper to taste.
6. Fold the other half of the tortilla over the filling to create a wrap.
7. Repeat with the second tortilla and remaining ingredients.
8. If desired, heat the wraps in the skillet for an additional 1-2 minutes on each side until the cheese is melted and the wrap is warmed through.
9. Slice each wrap in half and serve with salsa on the side if desired.
10. Enjoy your tasty and satisfying turkey and cheese breakfast wrap!

> **Nutritional Info:**
> **Calories: 300 | Protein: 18g | Carbohydrates: 25g | Fat: 15g | Fiber: 6g**

GASTRIC BYPASS COOKBOOK FOR ALL STAGES

Recipe Name:_____

Date: / /   *Time:*_____

Rating: ☆ ☆ ☆ ☆ ☆

S/N	Ingredients	Adjustment

Cooking Experience: _____
_____
_____
_____

Notes:_____
_____
_____
_____
_____
_____
_____

Spinach and Feta Frittata

Prep Time: 10 minutes | Cooking Time: 20 minutes | Servings: 2

Ingredients:

- 4 large eggs
- 1/4 cup milk or unsweetened almond milk
- Salt and pepper, to taste
- 1 tablespoon olive oil
- 1 cup fresh spinach leaves
- 1/4 cup crumbled feta cheese
- 1/4 cup diced tomatoes
- 1/4 cup diced red bell pepper
- Fresh parsley for garnish (optional)

Method of Preparation:

1. Preheat the oven to 350°F (175°C).
2. In a mixing bowl, whisk together eggs, milk, salt, and pepper until well combined.
3. Heat olive oil in an oven-safe skillet over medium heat.
4. Add fresh spinach leaves to the skillet and cook for 1-2 minutes until wilted.
5. Pour the egg mixture evenly over the spinach in the skillet.
6. Sprinkle crumbled feta cheese, diced tomatoes, and diced red bell pepper over the egg mixture.
7. Cook for 3-4 minutes until the edges start to set.
8. Transfer the skillet to the preheated oven and bake for about 15-20 minutes until the frittata is set and golden brown on top.
9. Remove from the oven and let it cool slightly.
10. Garnish with fresh parsley if desired.
11. Slice the frittata into wedges and serve.
12. Enjoy your delicious and nutritious spinach and feta frittata!

Nutritional Info:
Calories: 250 | Protein: 15g | Carbohydrates: 5g | Fat: 18g |
Fiber: 2g

GASTRIC BYPASS COOKBOOK FOR ALL STAGES

Recipe Name:_____

Date: / /   *Time:*_____

Rating: ☆ ☆ ☆ ☆ ☆

S/N	Ingredients	Adjustment

Cooking Experience: _____

_____
_____
_____

Notes:_____

_____
_____
_____
_____
_____
_____

Breakfast Burrito

Prep Time: 10 minutes | Cooking Time: 10 minutes | Servings: 2

Ingredients:

- 4 large eggs
- Salt and pepper, to taste
- 2 whole grain tortillas
- 1/2 cup black beans, drained and rinsed
- 1/4 cup shredded cheddar cheese
- 1/4 cup salsa
- 1/4 avocado, sliced
- Fresh cilantro for garnish (optional)

Method of Preparation:

1. In a mixing bowl, beat the eggs until well combined. Season with salt and pepper.
2. Heat a non-stick skillet over medium heat.
3. Pour the beaten eggs into the skillet and cook, stirring occasionally, until scrambled and cooked through.
4. Warm the whole grain tortillas in the skillet for about 1 minute on each side.
5. Divide the scrambled eggs evenly between the tortillas.
6. Top each tortilla with black beans, shredded cheddar cheese, salsa, and sliced avocado.
7. Garnish with fresh cilantro if desired.
8. Roll up the tortillas to form burritos.
9. Serve immediately and enjoy your hearty breakfast burritos!

Nutritional Info:
Calories: 350 | Protein: 20g | Carbohydrates: 25g | Fat: 18g | Fiber: 8g

GASTRIC BYPASS COOKBOOK FOR ALL STAGES

Recipe Name:_____

Date: / /   *Time:*_____

Rating: ☆ ☆ ☆ ☆ ☆

S/N	Ingredients	Adjustment

Cooking Experience: _____

_____

_____

_____

Notes:_____

_____

_____

_____

_____

_____

_____

Smoked Salmon Bagel

Prep Time: 10 minutes | Cooking Time: 0 minutes | Servings: 2

Ingredients:

- 2 whole grain bagels, sliced and toasted
- 4 oz smoked salmon
- 1/4 cup cream cheese
- 1/4 red onion, thinly sliced
- 1 tablespoon capers
- Fresh dill for garnish (optional)
- Lemon wedges for serving (optional)

Method of Preparation:

1. Spread cream cheese evenly on the toasted bagel halves.
2. Top each bagel half with smoked salmon.
3. Garnish with thinly sliced red onion and capers.
4. Sprinkle fresh dill on top if desired.
5. Serve with lemon wedges on the side for squeezing over the smoked salmon.
6. Enjoy your delicious and satisfying smoked salmon bagels!

Nutritional Info:
Calories: 300 | Protein: 20g | Carbohydrates: 35g | Fat: 10g | Fiber: 6g

GASTRIC BYPASS COOKBOOK FOR ALL STAGES

Recipe Name:_____

Date: / /   *Time:*_____

Rating: ☆ ☆ ☆ ☆ ☆

S/N	Ingredients	Adjustment

Cooking Experience: _____
_____
_____
_____

Notes:_____
_____
_____
_____
_____
_____
_____

Veggie Breakfast Burrito Bowl

Prep Time: 10 minutes | Cooking Time: 10 minutes | Servings: 2

Ingredients:

- 4 large eggs
- Salt and pepper, to taste
- 1 tablespoon olive oil
- 1/2 cup black beans, drained and rinsed
- 1/2 cup diced tomatoes
- 1/2 avocado, sliced
- 1/4 cup shredded cheddar cheese
- 1/4 cup salsa
- Fresh cilantro for garnish (optional)

Method of Preparation:

1. In a mixing bowl, beat the eggs until well combined. Season with salt and pepper.
2. Heat olive oil in a non-stick skillet over medium heat.
3. Pour the beaten eggs into the skillet and cook, stirring occasionally, until scrambled and cooked through.
4. Divide the scrambled eggs evenly between two serving bowls.
5. Top each bowl with black beans, diced tomatoes, avocado slices, shredded cheddar cheese, and salsa.
6. Garnish with fresh cilantro if desired.
7. Serve immediately and enjoy your delicious and nutritious veggie breakfast burrito bowls!

Nutritional Info:
Calories: 350 | Protein: 20g | Carbohydrates: 25g | Fat: 18g | Fiber: 8g

GASTRIC BYPASS COOKBOOK FOR ALL STAGES

Recipe Name:_____

Date: / /   *Time:*_____

Rating: ☆ ☆ ☆ ☆ ☆

S/N	Ingredients	Adjustment

Cooking Experience: _____
_____
_____
_____

Notes:_____
_____
_____
_____
_____
_____
_____

Quinoa Breakfast Bowl

Prep Time: 10 minutes | Cooking Time: 15 minutes | Servings: 2

Ingredients:

- 1/2 cup quinoa, rinsed
- 1 cup water or low-sodium vegetable broth
- 4 large eggs
- Salt and pepper, to taste
- 1/2 avocado, sliced
- 1/2 cup cherry tomatoes, halved
- 1/4 cup crumbled feta cheese
- Fresh basil leaves for garnish (optional)

Method of Preparation:

1. In a medium saucepan, combine quinoa and water or vegetable broth.
2. Bring to a boil, then reduce heat to low, cover, and simmer for 15 minutes or until quinoa is cooked and liquid is absorbed.
3. While the quinoa is cooking, prepare the eggs. In a separate skillet, heat olive oil over medium heat. Crack the eggs into the skillet and cook to desired doneness, seasoning with salt and pepper.
4. Divide the cooked quinoa between two serving bowls.
5. Top each bowl with a cooked egg, avocado slices, cherry tomatoes, and crumbled feta cheese.
6. Garnish with fresh basil leaves if desired.
7. Serve hot and enjoy your nutritious quinoa breakfast bowl!

Nutritional Info:
Calories: 350 | Protein: 20g | Carbohydrates: 30g | Fat: 18g | Fiber: 6g

GASTRIC BYPASS COOKBOOK FOR ALL STAGES

Recipe Name:_____

Date: / /   *Time:*_____

Rating: ☆ ☆ ☆ ☆ ☆

S/N	Ingredients	Adjustment

Cooking Experience: _____
_____
_____
_____

Notes:_____
_____
_____
_____
_____
_____
_____

Banana Nut Oatmeal

Prep Time: 5 minutes | Cooking Time: 10 minutes | Servings: 2

Ingredients:

- 1 cup old-fashioned oats
- 2 cups water or milk of choice
- 1 ripe banana, mashed
- 1/4 cup chopped nuts (such as almonds, walnuts, or pecans)
- 1 tablespoon honey or maple syrup (optional)
- Pinch of cinnamon
- Pinch of salt
- Sliced banana and additional nuts for garnish (optional)

Method of Preparation:

1. In a medium saucepan, bring water or milk to a boil.
2. Stir in the old-fashioned oats, mashed banana, chopped nuts, honey or maple syrup (if using), cinnamon, and salt.
3. Reduce heat to low and simmer for about 5-7 minutes, stirring occasionally, until oats are cooked and mixture has thickened to desired consistency.
4. Remove from heat and let it sit for a minute or two to cool slightly.
5. Divide the banana nut oatmeal between two serving bowls.
6. Garnish with sliced banana and additional nuts if desired.
7. Serve hot and enjoy your comforting banana nut oatmeal!

Nutritional Info:
Calories: 300 | Protein: 10g | Carbohydrates: 40g | Fat: 12g |
Fiber: 6g

GASTRIC BYPASS COOKBOOK FOR ALL STAGES

Recipe Name:_____

Date: / /   *Time:*_____

Rating: ☆ ☆ ☆ ☆ ☆

S/N	Ingredients	Adjustment

Cooking Experience: _____
_____
_____
_____

Notes:_____
_____
_____
_____
_____
_____
_____

Lunch Recipes

Grilled Chicken Salad

Prep Time: 15 minutes | Cooking Time: 15 minutes | Servings: 2

Ingredients:

- 2 boneless, skinless chicken breasts (4 oz each)
- Salt and pepper, to taste
- 4 cups mixed salad greens
- 1/2 cup cherry tomatoes, halved
- 1/4 cup cucumber, sliced
- 1/4 cup bell peppers, sliced
- 2 tablespoons balsamic vinaigrette dressing
- 1 tablespoon olive oil

Method of Preparation:

1. Preheat the grill or grill pan over medium-high heat.
2. Season the chicken breasts with salt and pepper.
3. Grill the chicken breasts for about 6-7 minutes per side, or until they are cooked through and no longer pink in the center.
4. While the chicken is grilling, prepare the salad. In a large mixing bowl, toss together the mixed salad greens, cherry tomatoes, cucumber, and bell peppers.
5. Drizzle the salad with balsamic vinaigrette dressing and olive oil, and toss to coat evenly.
6. Once the chicken is cooked, remove it from the grill and let it rest for a few minutes.
7. Slice the grilled chicken breasts into thin strips.
8. Divide the salad between two plates and top each with sliced grilled chicken.
9. Serve immediately and enjoy your delicious and nutritious grilled chicken salad!

Nutritional Info:
Calories: 300 | Protein: 25g | Carbohydrates: 10g | Fat: 15g |
Fiber: 4g

GASTRIC BYPASS COOKBOOK FOR ALL STAGES

Recipe Name:_____

Date: / /   *Time:*_____

Rating: ☆ ☆ ☆ ☆ ☆

S/N	Ingredients	Adjustment

Cooking Experience: _____
_____
_____
_____

Notes:_____
_____
_____
_____
_____
_____
_____

Turkey and Avocado Wrap

Prep Time: 10 minutes | Cooking Time: 0 minutes | Servings: 2

Ingredients:

- 4 large whole grain tortillas
- 8 slices turkey breast
- 1 avocado, sliced
- 1/2 cup mixed greens
- 2 tablespoons hummus
- Salt and pepper, to taste

Method of Preparation:

1. Lay out the tortillas on a flat surface.
2. Spread 1/2 tablespoon of hummus evenly over each tortilla.
3. Layer two slices of turkey breast, avocado slices, and mixed greens on each tortilla.
4. Season with salt and pepper to taste.
5. Roll up each tortilla tightly to form a wrap.
6. Slice each wrap in half diagonally.
7. Serve immediately and enjoy your flavorful and satisfying turkey and avocado wraps!

Nutritional Info:
Calories: 320 | Protein: 20g | Carbohydrates: 30g | Fat: 15g | Fiber: 8g

GASTRIC BYPASS COOKBOOK FOR ALL STAGES

Recipe Name:_____

Date: / /   *Time:*_____

Rating: ☆ ☆ ☆ ☆ ☆

S/N	Ingredients	Adjustment

Cooking Experience: _____
_____
_____
_____

Notes:_____
_____
_____
_____
_____
_____
_____

Salmon Quinoa Bowl

Prep Time: 10 minutes | Cooking Time: 20 minutes | Servings: 2

Ingredients:

- 2 salmon fillets (4 oz each)
- Salt and pepper, to taste
- 1 cup cooked quinoa
- 1 cup steamed broccoli florets
- 1/2 cup cherry tomatoes, halved
- 1/4 cup diced red onion
- 2 tablespoons chopped fresh parsley
- 1 tablespoon olive oil
- 1 tablespoon lemon juice

Method of Preparation:

1. Preheat the oven to 400°F (200°C).
2. Season the salmon fillets with salt and pepper and place them on a baking sheet lined with parchment paper.
3. Bake the salmon in the preheated oven for 12-15 minutes, or until cooked through and flaky.
4. While the salmon is baking, prepare the quinoa according to package instructions.
5. In a large mixing bowl, combine the cooked quinoa, steamed broccoli florets, cherry tomatoes, diced red onion, chopped parsley, olive oil, and lemon juice. Toss to combine.
6. Once the salmon is cooked, remove it from the oven and let it cool slightly.
7. Divide the quinoa mixture between two bowls and top each with a baked salmon fillet.
8. Serve immediately and enjoy your nutritious salmon quinoa bowls!

> ### *Nutritional Info:*
> *Calories: 350 | Protein: 25g | Carbohydrates: 25g | Fat: 18g |*
> *Fiber: 6g*

GASTRIC BYPASS COOKBOOK FOR ALL STAGES

Recipe Name:_____

Date: / /   *Time:*_____

Rating: ☆ ☆ ☆ ☆ ☆

S/N	Ingredients	Adjustment

Cooking Experience: _____
_____
_____
_____

Notes:_____
_____
_____
_____
_____
_____
_____

Turkey and Vegetable Stir-Fry

Prep Time: 15 minutes | Cooking Time: 15 minutes | Servings: 2

Ingredients:

- 8 oz turkey breast, thinly sliced
- Salt and pepper, to taste
- 2 tablespoons soy sauce
- 1 tablespoon hoisin sauce
- 1 tablespoon olive oil
- 1 cup mixed vegetables (such as bell peppers, broccoli, carrots)
- 2 cloves garlic, minced
- 1 teaspoon grated ginger
- Cooked brown rice or quinoa, for serving

Method of Preparation:

1. Season the thinly sliced turkey breast with salt and pepper.
2. In a small bowl, whisk together soy sauce and hoisin sauce. Set aside.
3. Heat olive oil in a large skillet or wok over medium-high heat.
4. Add the seasoned turkey breast slices to the skillet and stir-fry for 2-3 minutes until browned and cooked through. Remove from the skillet and set aside.
5. In the same skillet, add the mixed vegetables and stir-fry for 3-4 minutes until they are tender-crisp.
6. Add minced garlic and grated ginger to the skillet and stir-fry for another 1-2 minutes until fragrant.
7. Return the cooked turkey breast slices to the skillet.
8. Pour the soy sauce and hoisin sauce mixture over the turkey and vegetables. Stir to coat evenly and cook for an additional 1-2 minutes.

9. Serve the turkey and vegetable stir-fry over cooked brown rice or quinoa.
10. Enjoy your flavorful and satisfying stir-fry!

> ***Nutritional Info:***
> ***Calories: 320 | Protein: 25g | Carbohydrates: 20g | Fat: 15g | Fiber: 4g***

GASTRIC BYPASS COOKBOOK FOR ALL STAGES

Recipe Name:_____

Date: / /   *Time:*_____

Rating: ☆ ☆ ☆ ☆ ☆

S/N	Ingredients	Adjustment

Cooking Experience: _____

_____

_____

_____

Notes:_____

_____

_____

_____

_____

_____

_____

Quinoa and Black Bean Salad

Prep Time: 15 minutes | Cooking Time: 15 minutes | Servings: 2

Ingredients:

- 1/2 cup uncooked quinoa
- 1 cup water or vegetable broth
- 1 can (15 oz) black beans, drained and rinsed
- 1/2 cup corn kernels (fresh, canned, or frozen)
- 1/4 cup diced red bell pepper
- 1/4 cup diced red onion
- 1/4 cup chopped fresh cilantro
- Juice of 1 lime
- 2 tablespoons olive oil
- Salt and pepper, to taste
- **Optional toppings:** avocado slices, cherry tomatoes, shredded cheese

Method of Preparation:

1. Rinse the quinoa under cold water using a fine mesh sieve.
2. In a medium saucepan, bring the water or vegetable broth to a boil. Add the quinoa, reduce heat to low, cover, and simmer for 15 minutes or until all liquid is absorbed.
3. Fluff the cooked quinoa with a fork and transfer it to a large mixing bowl.
4. Add the black beans, corn kernels, diced red bell pepper, diced red onion, and chopped fresh cilantro to the bowl with the quinoa.
5. In a small bowl, whisk together the lime juice, olive oil, salt, and pepper to make the dressing.
6. Pour the dressing over the quinoa mixture and toss to combine until everything is evenly coated.
7. Divide the quinoa and black bean salad between two serving plates.

8. If desired, top each serving with avocado slices, cherry tomatoes, and shredded cheese.
9. Serve immediately and enjoy your refreshing quinoa and black bean salad!

Nutritional Info:
Calories: 320 | Protein: 12g | Carbohydrates: 45g | Fat: 10g | Fiber: 10g

GASTRIC BYPASS COOKBOOK FOR ALL STAGES

Recipe Name:_____

Date: / /   *Time:*_____

Rating: ☆ ☆ ☆ ☆ ☆

S/N	Ingredients	Adjustment

Cooking Experience: _____
_____
_____
_____

Notes:_____
_____
_____
_____
_____
_____
_____
_____

Greek Chicken Pita Pockets

Prep Time: 20 minutes | Cooking Time: 15 minutes | Servings: 2

Ingredients:

- 2 boneless, skinless chicken breasts (4 oz each)
- 1 tablespoon olive oil
- 1 teaspoon dried oregano
- 1/2 teaspoon garlic powder
- Salt and pepper, to taste
- 2 whole wheat pita pockets
- 1/2 cup Greek yogurt
- 1/4 cup diced cucumber
- 1/4 cup diced tomato
- 1/4 cup sliced red onion
- 2 tablespoons crumbled feta cheese
- Fresh parsley for garnish (optional)

Method of Preparation:

1. Preheat the grill or grill pan over medium-high heat.
2. Rub the chicken breasts with olive oil, dried oregano, garlic powder, salt, and pepper.
3. Grill the chicken breasts for 6-7 minutes per side, or until they are cooked through and no longer pink in the center.
4. While the chicken is grilling, warm the pita pockets according to package instructions.
5. In a small bowl, combine the Greek yogurt, diced cucumber, and diced tomato to make the tzatziki sauce.
6. Once the chicken is cooked, let it rest for a few minutes, then slice it into thin strips.
7. Cut the warm pita pockets in half and gently open each half to form a pocket.
8. Stuff each pita pocket with sliced grilled chicken, sliced red onion, and crumbled feta cheese.

9. Drizzle with tzatziki sauce and garnish with fresh parsley if desired.
10. Serve immediately and enjoy your delicious Greek chicken pita pockets!

Nutritional Info:
Calories: 350 | Protein: 25g | Carbohydrates: 30g | Fat: 15g |
Fiber: 6g

GASTRIC BYPASS COOKBOOK FOR ALL STAGES

Recipe Name:_____

Date: / /   *Time:*_____

Rating: ☆ ☆ ☆ ☆ ☆

S/N	Ingredients	Adjustment

Cooking Experience: _____
_____
_____
_____

Notes:_____
_____
_____
_____
_____
_____
_____

Turkey and Veggie Stir-Fry

Prep Time: 15 minutes | Cooking Time: 15 minutes | Servings: 2

Ingredients:

- 8 oz turkey breast, thinly sliced
- Salt and pepper, to taste
- 1 tablespoon olive oil
- 2 cups mixed vegetables (such as bell peppers, broccoli, carrots)
- 2 cloves garlic, minced
- 1 teaspoon grated ginger
- 2 tablespoons low-sodium soy sauce
- 1 tablespoon hoisin sauce
- Cooked brown rice or quinoa, for serving

Method of Preparation:

1. Season the thinly sliced turkey breast with salt and pepper.
2. Heat olive oil in a large skillet or wok over medium-high heat.
3. Add the seasoned turkey breast slices to the skillet and stir-fry for 2-3 minutes until browned and cooked through. Remove from the skillet and set aside.
4. In the same skillet, add the mixed vegetables and stir-fry for 3-4 minutes until they are tender-crisp.
5. Add minced garlic and grated ginger to the skillet and stir-fry for another 1-2 minutes until fragrant.
6. Return the cooked turkey breast slices to the skillet.
7. In a small bowl, mix together soy sauce and hoisin sauce. Pour the sauce over the turkey and vegetables. Stir to coat evenly and cook for an additional 1-2 minutes.
8. Serve the turkey and vegetable stir-fry over cooked brown rice or quinoa.
9. Enjoy your flavorful and satisfying stir-fry!

Nutritional Info:
Calories: 320 | Protein: 25g | Carbohydrates: 20g | Fat: 15g |
Fiber: 4g

GASTRIC BYPASS COOKBOOK FOR ALL STAGES

Recipe Name:_____

Date: / /   *Time:*____

Rating: ☆ ☆ ☆ ☆ ☆

S/N	Ingredients	Adjustment

Cooking Experience: _____

_____

_____

_____

Notes:_____

_____

_____

_____

_____

_____

_____

Caprese Chicken Salad

Prep Time: 10 minutes | Cooking Time: 15 minutes | Servings: 2

Ingredients:

- 2 boneless, skinless chicken breasts (4 oz each)
- Salt and pepper, to taste
- 1 tablespoon olive oil
- 1 cup cherry tomatoes, halved
- 1/2 cup fresh mozzarella balls, halved
- 1/4 cup fresh basil leaves, torn
- Balsamic glaze, for drizzling
- Mixed greens, for serving

Method of Preparation:

1. Season the chicken breasts with salt and pepper.
2. Heat olive oil in a skillet over medium-high heat.
3. Add the seasoned chicken breasts to the skillet and cook for 6-7 minutes per side, or until they are cooked through and no longer pink in the center.
4. While the chicken is cooking, prepare the salad. In a large mixing bowl, combine cherry tomatoes, fresh mozzarella balls, and torn basil leaves.
5. Once the chicken is cooked, let it rest for a few minutes, then slice it into thin strips.
6. Add the sliced chicken to the salad bowl and toss to combine.
7. Divide mixed greens between two plates and top with the caprese chicken salad.
8. Drizzle with balsamic glaze before serving.
9. Enjoy your delicious and fresh caprese chicken salad!

Nutritional Info:
Calories: 320 | Protein: 25g | Carbohydrates: 10g | Fat: 18g |
Fiber: 2g

GASTRIC BYPASS COOKBOOK FOR ALL STAGES

Recipe Name:_____

Date: / /   *Time:*_____

Rating: ☆ ☆ ☆ ☆ ☆

S/N	Ingredients	Adjustment

Cooking Experience: _____
_____
_____
_____

Notes:_____
_____
_____
_____
_____
_____
_____

Turkey and Quinoa Stuffed Bell Peppers

Prep Time: 20 minutes | Cooking Time: 40 minutes | Servings: 2

Ingredients:

- 2 large bell peppers, halved and seeds removed
- 1/2 cup uncooked quinoa
- 1 cup water or low-sodium chicken broth
- 8 oz lean ground turkey
- 1/4 cup diced onion
- 1/4 cup diced tomatoes
- 1/4 cup diced zucchini
- 1/4 cup diced mushrooms
- 1/4 cup shredded mozzarella cheese
- 1 teaspoon Italian seasoning
- Salt and pepper, to taste
- Fresh parsley for garnish (optional)

Method of Preparation:

1. Preheat the oven to 375°F (190°C).
2. In a medium saucepan, bring water or chicken broth to a boil. Add quinoa, reduce heat to low, cover, and simmer for 15-20 minutes or until quinoa is cooked and liquid is absorbed.
3. In a skillet, cook ground turkey over medium heat until browned. Add diced onion, tomatoes, zucchini, and mushrooms. Cook until vegetables are tender.
4. Stir in cooked quinoa, Italian seasoning, salt, and pepper. Mix well.
5. Fill each bell pepper half with the turkey and quinoa mixture.
6. Place stuffed bell peppers in a baking dish. Cover with aluminum foil and bake for 25-30 minutes.

7. Remove foil, sprinkle shredded mozzarella cheese on top of each stuffed bell pepper, and bake for an additional 5-10 minutes or until cheese is melted and bubbly.
8. Garnish with fresh parsley before serving.
9. Enjoy your flavorful turkey and quinoa stuffed bell peppers!

Nutritional Info:
Calories: 350 | Protein: 25g | Carbohydrates: 30g | Fat: 15g | Fiber: 6g

GASTRIC BYPASS COOKBOOK FOR ALL STAGES

Recipe Name:_____

Date: / /   *Time:*_____

Rating: ☆ ☆ ☆ ☆ ☆

S/N	Ingredients	Adjustment

Cooking Experience: _____
_____
_____
_____

Notes:_____
_____
_____
_____
_____
_____
_____

Chicken Caesar Salad

Prep Time: 15 minutes | Cooking Time: 15 minutes | Servings: 2

Ingredients:

- 2 boneless, skinless chicken breasts (4 oz each)
- Salt and pepper, to taste
- 2 tablespoons olive oil, divided
- 4 cups chopped romaine lettuce
- 1/4 cup grated Parmesan cheese
- 1/4 cup whole grain croutons
- Caesar dressing (store-bought or homemade)
- Lemon wedges for serving (optional)

Method of Preparation:

1. Season the chicken breasts with salt and pepper.
2. Heat 1 tablespoon of olive oil in a skillet over medium-high heat.
3. Add the seasoned chicken breasts to the skillet and cook for 6-7 minutes per side, or until they are cooked through and no longer pink in the center.
4. Remove the chicken from the skillet and let it rest for a few minutes. Then slice it into thin strips.
5. In a large mixing bowl, combine chopped romaine lettuce, grated Parmesan cheese, and whole grain croutons.
6. Add the sliced chicken to the salad bowl.
7. Drizzle Caesar dressing over the salad and toss to coat evenly.
8. Divide the chicken Caesar salad between two plates.
9. Serve with lemon wedges on the side for squeezing over the salad if desired.
10. Enjoy your classic and satisfying chicken Caesar salad!

Nutritional Info:
Calories: 320 | Protein: 25g | Carbohydrates: 15g | Fat: 18g | Fiber: 4g

GASTRIC BYPASS COOKBOOK FOR ALL STAGES

Recipe Name:_____

Date: / /   *Time:*_____

Rating: ☆ ☆ ☆ ☆ ☆

S/N	Ingredients	Adjustment

Cooking Experience: _____
_____
_____
_____

Notes:_____
_____
_____
_____
_____
_____
_____

Dinner Recipes
Baked Lemon Herb Salmon

Prep Time: 10 minutes | Cooking Time: 15 minutes | Servings: 2

Ingredients:

- 2 salmon fillets (4 oz each)
- Salt and pepper, to taste
- 1 tablespoon olive oil
- 1 lemon, thinly sliced
- 2 cloves garlic, minced
- 1 teaspoon dried thyme
- 1 teaspoon dried rosemary
- Fresh parsley for garnish (optional)

Method of Preparation:

1. Preheat the oven to 400°F (200°C). Line a baking sheet with parchment paper.
2. Place the salmon fillets on the prepared baking sheet.
3. Season the salmon fillets with salt and pepper.
4. Drizzle olive oil over the salmon fillets and rub to coat evenly.
5. Arrange lemon slices over the top of each salmon fillet.
6. Sprinkle minced garlic, dried thyme, and dried rosemary over the lemon slices.
7. Bake in the preheated oven for 12-15 minutes, or until the salmon is cooked through and flakes easily with a fork.
8. Remove from the oven and garnish with fresh parsley before serving.
9. Serve immediately and enjoy your flavorful baked lemon herb salmon!

Nutritional Info: Calories: 300 | Protein: 25g | Carbohydrates: 5g | Fat: 18g | Fiber: 1g

GASTRIC BYPASS COOKBOOK FOR ALL STAGES

Recipe Name:_____

Date: / /   *Time:*_____

Rating: ☆ ☆ ☆ ☆ ☆

S/N	Ingredients	Adjustment

Cooking Experience: _____
_____
_____
_____

Notes:_____
_____
_____
_____
_____
_____
_____
_____

Grilled Chicken and Vegetable Skewers

Prep Time: 20 minutes | Cooking Time: 10 minutes | Servings: 2

Ingredients:

- 2 boneless, skinless chicken breasts (4 oz each), cut into cubes
- Salt and pepper, to taste
- 1 bell pepper, cut into chunks
- 1 zucchini, sliced
- 1 red onion, cut into chunks
- 8 cherry tomatoes
- 1 tablespoon olive oil
- 1 teaspoon Italian seasoning
- Wooden skewers, soaked in water for 30 minutes

Method of Preparation:

1. Preheat the grill or grill pan over medium-high heat.
2. Season the chicken breast cubes with salt, pepper, and Italian seasoning.
3. Thread the marinated chicken, bell pepper chunks, zucchini slices, red onion chunks, and cherry tomatoes onto the soaked wooden skewers, alternating between ingredients.
4. Drizzle olive oil over the assembled skewers.
5. Grill the skewers for 4-5 minutes on each side, or until the chicken is cooked through and the vegetables are tender.
6. Remove the skewers from the grill and let them rest for a few minutes.
7. Serve the grilled chicken and vegetable skewers hot.
8. Enjoy your delicious and colorful meal!

Nutritional Info: Calories: 280 | Protein: 25g | Carbohydrates: 15g | Fat: 12g | Fiber: 4g

GASTRIC BYPASS COOKBOOK FOR ALL STAGES

Recipe Name:_____

Date: / /   *Time:*_____

Rating: ☆ ☆ ☆ ☆ ☆

S/N	Ingredients	Adjustment

Cooking Experience: _____
_____
_____
_____

Notes:_____
_____
_____
_____
_____
_____
_____

Beef and Vegetable Stir-Fry

Prep Time: 15 minutes | Cooking Time: 15 minutes | Servings: 2

Ingredients:

- 8 oz beef sirloin, thinly sliced
- Salt and pepper, to taste
- 1 tablespoon olive oil
- 2 cups mixed vegetables (such as bell peppers, broccoli, carrots)
- 2 cloves garlic, minced
- 1 teaspoon grated ginger
- 2 tablespoons low-sodium soy sauce
- 1 tablespoon hoisin sauce
- Cooked brown rice or quinoa, for serving

Method of Preparation:

1. Season the thinly sliced beef sirloin with salt and pepper.
2. Heat olive oil in a large skillet or wok over medium-high heat.
3. Add the seasoned beef slices to the skillet and stir-fry for 2-3 minutes until browned.
4. Remove the beef from the skillet and set aside.
5. In the same skillet, add the mixed vegetables and stir-fry for 3-4 minutes until they are tender-crisp.
6. Add minced garlic and grated ginger to the skillet and stir-fry for another 1-2 minutes until fragrant.
7. Return the cooked beef slices to the skillet.
8. In a small bowl, mix together soy sauce and hoisin sauce. Pour the sauce over the beef and vegetables. Stir to coat evenly and cook for an additional 1-2 minutes.
9. Serve the beef and vegetable stir-fry over cooked brown rice or quinoa.
10. Enjoy your flavorful and satisfying stir-fry!

Nutritional Info:
Calories: 330 | Protein: 25g | Carbohydrates: 20g | Fat: 15g |
Fiber: 4g

GASTRIC BYPASS COOKBOOK FOR ALL STAGES

Recipe Name:_____

Date: / /   *Time:*_____

Rating: ☆ ☆ ☆ ☆ ☆

S/N	Ingredients	Adjustment

Cooking Experience: _____

_____

_____

_____

Notes:_____

_____

_____

_____

_____

_____

_____

Shrimp and Asparagus Pasta

Prep Time: 10 minutes | Cooking Time: 20 minutes | Servings: 2

Ingredients:
- 6 oz whole wheat spaghetti
- 8 oz shrimp, peeled and deveined
- Salt and pepper, to taste
- 1 tablespoon olive oil
- 2 cloves garlic, minced
- 1 bunch asparagus, trimmed and cut into bite-sized pieces
- 1/4 cup cherry tomatoes, halved
- 2 tablespoons grated Parmesan cheese
- Fresh parsley for garnish (optional)

Method of Preparation:
1. Cook the whole wheat spaghetti according to package instructions until al dente. Drain and set aside.
2. Season the shrimp with salt and pepper.
3. Heat olive oil in a large skillet over medium heat. Add minced garlic and cook for 1 minute until fragrant.
4. Add the seasoned shrimp to the skillet and cook for 2-3 minutes on each side until pink and cooked through.
5. Remove the cooked shrimp from the skillet and set aside.
6. In the same skillet, add the asparagus pieces and cherry tomatoes. Cook for 4-5 minutes until the vegetables are tender.
7. Return the cooked shrimp to the skillet.
8. Add the cooked whole wheat spaghetti to the skillet and toss to combine with the shrimp and vegetables.
9. Divide the shrimp and asparagus pasta between two serving plates.
10. Garnish with grated Parmesan cheese and fresh parsley, if desired.

11. Serve immediately and enjoy your delicious shrimp and asparagus pasta!

> **Nutritional Info:**
> **Calories: 350 | Protein: 30g | Carbohydrates: 40g | Fat: 10g | Fiber: 8g**

GASTRIC BYPASS COOKBOOK FOR ALL STAGES

Recipe Name:_____

Date: / /   *Time:*____

Rating: ☆ ☆ ☆ ☆ ☆

S/N	Ingredients	Adjustment

Cooking Experience: _____
_____
_____
_____

Notes:_____
_____
_____
_____
_____
_____
_____
_____

Baked Chicken Parmesan

Prep Time: 15 minutes | Cooking Time: 25 minutes | Servings: 2

Ingredients:

- 2 boneless, skinless chicken breasts (4 oz each)
- Salt and pepper, to taste
- 1/2 cup whole wheat breadcrumbs
- 1/4 cup grated Parmesan cheese
- 1 teaspoon Italian seasoning
- 1 egg, beaten
- 1 cup marinara sauce
- 1/2 cup shredded mozzarella cheese
- Fresh basil leaves for garnish (optional)

Method of Preparation:

1. Preheat the oven to 400°F (200°C). Line a baking sheet with parchment paper.
2. Season the chicken breasts with salt and pepper.
3. In a shallow dish, combine whole wheat breadcrumbs, grated Parmesan cheese, and Italian seasoning.
4. Dip each chicken breast into the beaten egg, then coat with the breadcrumb mixture.
5. Place the coated chicken breasts on the prepared baking sheet.
6. Bake in the preheated oven for 20 minutes.
7. Remove the chicken from the oven and spoon marinara sauce over each chicken breast.
8. Sprinkle shredded mozzarella cheese on top of the marinara sauce.
9. Return the chicken to the oven and bake for an additional 5 minutes, or until the cheese is melted and bubbly.
10. Garnish with fresh basil leaves before serving.
11. Serve hot and enjoy your baked chicken Parmesan!

Nutritional Info:
Calories: 350 | Protein: 30g | Carbohydrates: 20g | Fat: 15g |
Fiber: 3g

GASTRIC BYPASS COOKBOOK FOR ALL STAGES

Recipe Name:_____

Date: / /   *Time:*_____

Rating: ☆ ☆ ☆ ☆ ☆

S/N	Ingredients	Adjustment

Cooking Experience: _____
_____
_____
_____

Notes:_____
_____
_____
_____
_____
_____
_____
_____

Turkey and Quinoa Stuffed Bell Peppers

Prep Time: 20 minutes | Cooking Time: 40 minutes | Servings: 2

Ingredients:

- 2 large bell peppers, halved and seeds removed
- 1/2 cup uncooked quinoa
- 1 cup water or low-sodium chicken broth
- 8 oz lean ground turkey
- 1/4 cup diced onion
- 1/4 cup diced tomatoes
- 1/4 cup diced zucchini
- 1/4 cup diced mushrooms
- 1/4 cup shredded mozzarella cheese
- 1 teaspoon Italian seasoning
- Salt and pepper, to taste
- Fresh parsley for garnish (optional)

Method of Preparation:

1. Preheat the oven to 375°F (190°C).
2. In a medium saucepan, bring water or chicken broth to a boil. Add quinoa, reduce heat to low, cover, and simmer for 15-20 minutes or until quinoa is cooked and liquid is absorbed.
3. In a skillet, cook ground turkey over medium heat until browned. Add diced onion, tomatoes, zucchini, and mushrooms. Cook until vegetables are tender.
4. Stir in cooked quinoa, Italian seasoning, salt, and pepper. Mix well.
5. Fill each bell pepper half with the turkey and quinoa mixture.
6. Place stuffed bell peppers in a baking dish. Cover with aluminum foil and bake for 25-30 minutes.

7. Remove foil, sprinkle shredded mozzarella cheese on top of each stuffed bell pepper, and bake for an additional 5-10 minutes or until cheese is melted and bubbly.
8. Garnish with fresh parsley before serving.
9. Enjoy your flavorful turkey and quinoa stuffed bell peppers!

Nutritional Info:
Calories: 320 | Protein: 25g | Carbohydrates: 30g | Fat: 15g | Fiber: 6g

GASTRIC BYPASS COOKBOOK FOR ALL STAGES

Recipe Name:_____

Date: / /   *Time:*_____

Rating: ☆ ☆ ☆ ☆ ☆

S/N	Ingredients	Adjustment

Cooking Experience: _____
_____
_____
_____

Notes:_____
_____
_____
_____
_____
_____
_____

Baked Garlic Butter Salmon with Asparagus

Prep Time: 10 minutes | Cooking Time: 20 minutes | Servings: 2

Ingredients:

- 2 salmon fillets (4 oz each)
- Salt and pepper, to taste
- 2 tablespoons unsalted butter, melted
- 2 cloves garlic, minced
- 1 tablespoon fresh lemon juice
- 1 bunch asparagus, trimmed
- 1 tablespoon olive oil
- Lemon slices for garnish (optional)

Method of Preparation:

1. Preheat the oven to 400°F (200°C). Line a baking sheet with parchment paper.
2. Season the salmon fillets with salt and pepper, then place them on the prepared baking sheet.
3. In a small bowl, mix together melted butter, minced garlic, and fresh lemon juice.
4. Brush the garlic butter mixture over the salmon fillets.
5. Toss the trimmed asparagus with olive oil, salt, and pepper in a separate bowl.
6. Arrange the asparagus around the salmon fillets on the baking sheet.
7. Bake in the preheated oven for 15-20 minutes, or until the salmon is cooked through and flakes easily with a fork, and the asparagus is tender.
8. Remove from the oven and garnish with lemon slices, if desired.
9. Serve hot and enjoy your delicious baked garlic butter salmon with asparagus!

Nutritional Info:
Calories: 320 | Protein: 25g | Carbohydrates: 6g | Fat: 22g | Fiber: 3g

GASTRIC BYPASS COOKBOOK FOR ALL STAGES

Recipe Name:_____

Date: / /   *Time:*_____

Rating: ☆ ☆ ☆ ☆ ☆

S/N	Ingredients	Adjustment

Cooking Experience: _____
_____
_____
_____

Notes:_____
_____
_____
_____
_____
_____
_____
_____

Turkey Taco Lettuce Wraps

Prep Time: 15 minutes | Cooking Time: 15 minutes | Servings: 2

Ingredients:

- 8 oz lean ground turkey
- 1 tablespoon olive oil
- 1/2 cup diced onion
- 1/2 cup diced bell pepper
- 2 cloves garlic, minced
- 1 tablespoon chili powder
- 1 teaspoon ground cumin
- 1/2 teaspoon paprika
- Salt and pepper, to taste
- 1/2 cup tomato sauce
- Iceberg lettuce leaves, for wrapping
- **Optional toppings:** diced tomato, sliced avocado, shredded cheese, Greek yogurt

Method of Preparation:

1. Heat olive oil in a skillet over medium heat. Add diced onion and bell pepper, and cook until softened, about 5 minutes.
2. Add minced garlic and cook for another minute until fragrant.
3. Add ground turkey to the skillet and cook until browned, breaking it apart with a spatula as it cooks.
4. Stir in chili powder, cumin, paprika, salt, and pepper.
5. Pour tomato sauce into the skillet and stir to combine. Cook for an additional 5 minutes until heated through.
6. Spoon the turkey taco mixture onto iceberg lettuce leaves.
7. Top with optional toppings such as diced tomato, sliced avocado, shredded cheese, and Greek yogurt.
8. Serve immediately and enjoy your tasty turkey taco lettuce wraps!

GASTRIC BYPASS COOKBOOK FOR ALL STAGES

> **Nutritional Info:**
> **Calories: 280 | Protein: 25g | Carbohydrates: 10g | Fat: 15g | Fiber: 3g**

GASTRIC BYPASS COOKBOOK FOR ALL STAGES

Recipe Name:_____

Date: / /   *Time:*_____

Rating: ☆ ☆ ☆ ☆ ☆

S/N	Ingredients	Adjustment

Cooking Experience: _____

_____

_____

_____

Notes:_____

_____

_____

_____

_____

_____

_____

Grilled Lemon Herb Chicken Breast

Prep Time: 10 minutes | Cooking Time: 15 minutes | Servings: 2

Ingredients:

- 2 boneless, skinless chicken breasts (4 oz each)
- Salt and pepper, to taste
- 2 tablespoons olive oil
- Zest and juice of 1 lemon
- 2 cloves garlic, minced
- 1 teaspoon dried thyme
- 1 teaspoon dried rosemary
- Fresh parsley for garnish (optional)

Method of Preparation:

1. Preheat the grill to medium-high heat.
2. Season the chicken breasts with salt and pepper.
3. In a small bowl, whisk together olive oil, lemon zest, lemon juice, minced garlic, dried thyme, and dried rosemary.
4. Brush the lemon herb mixture over both sides of the chicken breasts.
5. Place the chicken breasts on the preheated grill and cook for 6-8 minutes on each side, or until cooked through and no longer pink in the center.
6. Remove the chicken from the grill and let it rest for a few minutes.
7. Garnish with fresh parsley before serving.
8. Serve hot and enjoy your delicious grilled lemon herb chicken breast!

Nutritional Info:
Calories: 280 | Protein: 25g | Carbohydrates: 2g | Fat: 18g |
Fiber: 1g

GASTRIC BYPASS COOKBOOK FOR ALL STAGES

Recipe Name:_____

Date: / /   *Time:*_____

Rating: ☆ ☆ ☆ ☆ ☆

S/N	Ingredients	Adjustment

Cooking Experience: _____

_____

_____

_____

Notes:_____

_____

_____

_____

_____

_____

_____

Baked Turkey and Vegetable Casserole

Prep Time: 20 minutes | Cooking Time: 30 minutes | Servings: 2

Ingredients:

- 8 oz lean ground turkey
- Salt and pepper, to taste
- 1 tablespoon olive oil
- 1/2 cup diced onion
- 1/2 cup diced bell pepper
- 1/2 cup diced zucchini
- 1/2 cup diced tomatoes
- 1/2 cup cooked quinoa
- 1/4 cup shredded mozzarella cheese
- 1/4 cup grated Parmesan cheese
- 1 teaspoon Italian seasoning
- Fresh parsley for garnish (optional)

Method of Preparation:

1. Preheat the oven to 375°F (190°C). Grease a baking dish with cooking spray.
2. In a skillet, heat olive oil over medium heat. Add diced onion, bell pepper, and zucchini. Cook until softened, about 5 minutes.
3. Add ground turkey to the skillet and cook until browned, breaking it apart with a spatula.
4. Season the turkey and vegetable mixture with salt, pepper, and Italian seasoning.
5. In a large mixing bowl, combine the cooked quinoa, diced tomatoes, and turkey and vegetable mixture.
6. Transfer the mixture to the greased baking dish and spread it out evenly.

7. Sprinkle shredded mozzarella cheese and grated Parmesan cheese over the top.
8. Bake in the preheated oven for 25-30 minutes, or until the cheese is melted and bubbly.
9. Garnish with fresh parsley before serving.
10. Serve hot and enjoy your flavorful baked turkey and vegetable casserole!

Nutritional Info:
Calories: 320 | Protein: 25g | Carbohydrates: 15g | Fat: 18g |
Fiber: 3g

GASTRIC BYPASS COOKBOOK FOR ALL STAGES

Recipe Name:_____

Date: / /   *Time:*_____

Rating: ☆ ☆ ☆ ☆ ☆

S/N	Ingredients	Adjustment

Cooking Experience: _____

_____

_____

_____

Notes:_____

_____

_____

_____

_____

_____

_____

GASTRIC BYPASS COOKBOOK FOR ALL STAGES

CHAPTER FIVE
Meal Planning and Portion Control

Meal planning and portion control are crucial aspects of maintaining a healthy diet, especially for individuals who have undergone gastric bypass surgery.

In this chapter, we will explore effective strategies for planning meals and snacks to ensure balanced nutrition, as well as provide guidelines and visual aids for estimating serving sizes to promote portion control.

Strategies for Planning Meals and Snacks

Prioritize Protein:
Protein is essential for tissue repair, muscle growth, and satiety. Aim to include a lean source of protein in each meal and snack to promote fullness and prevent muscle loss. Examples of protein-rich foods include poultry, fish, lean meats, eggs, dairy products, tofu, and legumes.

Incorporate Vegetables and Fruits:
Vegetables and fruits are rich in vitamins, minerals, fiber, and antioxidants, making them essential components of a balanced diet. Aim to fill half of your plate with non-starchy vegetables and include fruits as snacks or dessert options. Experiment with different colors and varieties to maximize nutrient intake.

Choose Whole Grains:

Whole grains provide complex carbohydrates, fiber, and essential nutrients. Opt for whole grain options such as brown rice, quinoa, whole wheat pasta, and whole grain bread to increase satiety and stabilize blood sugar levels. Limit refined grains and processed carbohydrates, which can lead to rapid spikes in blood sugar.

Include Healthy Fats:

Incorporate sources of healthy fats, such as avocados, nuts, seeds, olive oil, and fatty fish, into your meals and snacks. Healthy fats are important for nutrient absorption, brain function, and heart health. However, be mindful of portion sizes as fats are calorie-dense.

Plan Balanced Meals:

Aim to create balanced meals that contain a combination of protein, carbohydrates, and fats. This balance helps to provide sustained energy, regulate appetite, and prevent nutrient deficiencies. Use the plate method as a guide, dividing your plate into sections for protein, vegetables, fruits, and whole grains.

Prepare Meals in Advance:

Spend time each week planning and preparing meals in advance to streamline the cooking process and ensure healthy options are readily available. Batch cooking, portioning meals into containers, and utilizing slow cookers or Instant Pots can save time and promote consistency in eating habits.

Stay Hydrated:

Adequate hydration is essential for overall health and digestion. Aim to drink plenty of water throughout the day and limit sugary beverages and caffeinated drinks. Herbal teas, infused water, and low-calorie beverages can add variety to your hydration routine.

Portion Control Guidelines and Visual Aids

Use Portion Control Tools:

Invest in portion control tools such as measuring cups, spoons, and food scales to accurately measure serving sizes. These tools can help you become more aware of appropriate portion sizes and prevent overeating.

Follow Plate Portions:

Use the plate method as a visual guide for portion control. Fill half of your plate with non-starchy vegetables, one-quarter with lean protein, and one-quarter with whole grains or starchy vegetables. This method helps to ensure a balanced and satisfying meal.

Practice Mindful Eating:

Pay attention to hunger and fullness cues, and practice mindful eating to avoid mindless overeating. Eat slowly, savor each bite, and pause between bites to assess your level of hunger and satisfaction.

Understand Serving Sizes:

Familiarize yourself with standard serving sizes for common foods and food groups. For example, a serving of protein is typically 3-4 ounces, a serving of grains is one slice of bread or 1/2 cup cooked rice, and a serving of vegetables is 1 cup raw or 1/2 cup cooked.

Visualize Portions:

Use visual aids to estimate portion sizes when measuring tools are not available. For example, a serving of protein is roughly the size of a deck of cards, a serving of grains is about the size of a tennis ball, and a serving of fats is equivalent to the size of your thumb.

Practice Portion Distortion Awareness:

Be mindful of portion distortion, which occurs when large portion sizes become the norm. Restaurant portions and packaged foods often contain more calories and larger servings than necessary. Aim to split meals when dining out or portion out servings before eating.

Listen to Your Body:

Pay attention to how your body responds to different portion sizes and adjust accordingly. Focus on eating until you are satisfied rather than overly full, and practice moderation with indulgent foods.

Meal planning and portion control are essential strategies for promoting balanced nutrition, supporting weight management, and optimizing health outcomes after gastric bypass surgery. By prioritizing protein, incorporating a variety of nutrient-dense foods, and practicing portion control, individuals can create sustainable eating habits that contribute to long-term success and well-being.

CONCLUSION

Adopting a complete nutritional strategy is critical on the path to weight loss and increased health following gastric bypass surgery.

This cookbook, "Gastric Bypass Cookbook for All Stages: Quick and Easy Mouthwatering Recipes to Avoid Weight Gain at All Stages After Bariatric Surgery," is an invaluable resource for patients as they advance through the phases of recovery and dietary changes.

This book enables patients to achieve long-term success and optimal outcomes by providing tasty and nutritious recipes targeted to each step of the post-surgery journey, as well as crucial advice on meal planning, portion management, and balanced nutrition.

Gastric bypass surgery has several phases of recovery, each needing careful consideration of food choices and nutritional demands. Patients have distinct obstacles and chances for growth as they progress from liquid and pureed diets to soft foods and, eventually, conventional foods.

This cookbook recognizes the significance of guiding people through each stage, providing a broad selection of dishes that are both tasty and nutritious. Whether it's creamy protein drinks for the liquid diet phase, delicate turkey meatballs for the soft foods phase, or tasty grilled chicken for the regular foods phase, this book makes sure patients have access to meals that support healing and weight reduction.

At the core of this cookbook is a dedication to balanced nutrition. Each recipe is carefully designed to provide the nutrients required for maximum health and well-being.

By stressing lean meats, colorful fruits and vegetables, whole grains, and healthy fats, this book encourages readers to make nutritional choices that support their objectives.

Furthermore, the inclusion of meal planning tactics and portion management recommendations enables patients to take control of their eating habits and build a long-term approach to nutrition. Individuals may establish a healthy relationship with food and fuel their bodies for achievement by putting excellent foods first and practicing mindful eating.

This cookbook is more than simply a recipe collection; it is also a thorough instructional resource for both patients and healthcare professionals. Readers obtain vital insights into their own dietary needs and issues by reading extensive descriptions of gastric bypass surgery, the need of good nutrition after surgery, and practical recommendations for navigating meal choices.

This book empowers individuals by providing them with knowledge and insight, allowing them to make educated decisions about their health and take charge of their wellness path.

While gastric bypass surgery can be an effective strategy for weight loss and increased health, long-term success necessitates consistent focus and support.

This cookbook emphasizes the significance of creating a welcoming atmosphere for people on their post-surgery journey. This book is a reliable companion for patients as they navigate the ups and downs of weight loss and maintenance, offering a plethora of tasty recipes, practical advice, and inspiring ideas.

Whether celebrating achievements, overcoming setbacks, or seeking encouragement, this book may provide inspiration and insight every step of the journey.

As people begin their post-surgery journey, it's important to understand that improvement isn't always linear. There will be hurdles and barriers along the path, but with dedication, resilience, and the correct tools, success is achievable. This cookbook is more than simply a compilation of recipes; it's a road map for achieving long-term health and wellness.

Individuals may alter their life by embracing the ideas of balanced nutrition, portion management, and mindful eating.

The Gastric Bypass Cookbook for All Stages is more than simply a cookbook; it is also a transformational manual. This book enables people to take control of their health and reclaim their lives by providing a thorough approach to nutrition, practical recommendations, and tasty food ideas.

Whether you're starting your post-surgery journey or supporting someone who is, this cookbook will be your reliable companion on the road to long-term success. Together, we can work toward a healthier, happier future—one meal at a time.

Printed in Dunstable, United Kingdom